PAIN
RELIEF

PAIN RELIEF

Managing Chronic Pain through
Traditional, Holistic, and Eastern Practices

DAVID COSIO, PhD, ABPP

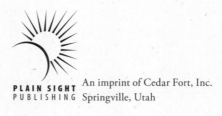

PLAIN SIGHT
PUBLISHING An imprint of Cedar Fort, Inc.
Springville, Utah

ISBN 13: 978-1-4621-2215-8

Published by Plain Sight Publishing, an imprint of Cedar Fort, Inc.
2373 W. 700 S., Springville, UT 84663
Distributed by Cedar Fort, Inc., www.cedarfort.com

LIBRARY OF CONGRESS CATALOGING-IN-PUBLICATION DATA

Names: Cosio, David, 1978- author.
Title: Pain relief : managing chronic pain through traditional, holistic, and eastern practices / David Cosio.
Description: Springville, Utah : Plain Sight Publishing, an imprint of Cedar Fort, Inc., [2018] | Includes bibliographical references and index.
Identifiers: LCCN 2018016870 (print) | LCCN 2018027866 (ebook) | ISBN 9781462129218 (epub, pdf, mobi) | ISBN 9781462122158 (perfect bound : alk. paper)
Subjects: LCSH: Pain--Treatment--Popular works.
Classification: LCC RB127 (ebook) | LCC RB127 .C695 2018 (print) | DDC 616/.0472--dc23
LC record available at https://lccn.loc.gov/2018016870

Cover design by Shawnda T. Craig
Cover design © 2018 Cedar Fort, Inc.
Edited by Deborah Spencer and Justin Greer
Typeset by Kaitlin Barwick

Printed in the United States of America

10 9 8 7 6 5 4 3 2 1

Printed on acid-free paper

Disclaimer

The views expressed by Dr. Cosio are based on his experience as a psychologist employed by the Veterans Administration. The views expressed do not necessarily represent those of the Department of Veterans Affairs or any other governmental agency.

Contents

Preface

I have been working in the field of pain management for the past ten years. Having been trained in clinical health psychology, I have learned about the skills I need in order to address the needs of people dealing with different health conditions. Perhaps the most difficult populace to work with is the chronic pain population. Not only do these people deal with a great deal of stigma, but now they are also faced with the repercussions of the opioid epidemic. Over the past decade, I have learned a lot about the different treatments that are available for pain management. I also have learned that most people who suffer from chronic pain do not have this information available to them. I truly believe that an informed patient is an empowered patient. This perspective led to the development of the *Pain Education School* program outlined in chapter 1. This program has been in existence for the past decade, and other models similar to it have been implemented in different hospital systems.

I came to write this book because I started doing speaking engagements across the country with providers who work with people who suffer from chronic pain. In these speaking engagements, I witnessed a need to share the information I gathered for the *Pain Education School* to these populations. This book is different from any other out on the book shelf in several different ways.

1. This book is a resource for not only those who suffer with chronic pain but also their families and healthcare providers.
2. This book can serve as a guide and supplement to the advice of the person's physician, whom you should continue to consult for individual medical problems.
3. This book includes information about interventional pain management procedures, medications, psychological treatments, physical therapies, and complementary and integrative approaches.
4. This book includes a section on lifestyle imbalances that are often ignored or taken for granted.
5. This book includes a section on how to empower providers and people with chronic pain and a section on coping with chronic pain. Often, similar books cover treatments but don't cover coping skills or vice versa.

Each chapter begins with *Questions for the Reader to Ponder*. These are questions that you will be able to answer once you have read the chapter. This section gives the reader an advanced look at what is covered in each chapter.

Every chapter has sections entitled *A Closer Look*. These sections give more detailed information about certain topics covered throughout the discussion in the chapter.

Several chapters have *Quick Guides*. These guides go into further detail about the treatments being outlined and frequently add additional information that is not offered in the discussion.

Several chapters have *A Patient Story*. These stories are used to illustrate common dilemmas faced by providers who work with people who have chronic pain. Often, these stories introduce other factors to consider that may have had an impact on the outcome.

The book is laid out in three general sections: pain education, assessment, and treatment. The objective is to put pain management into your hands.

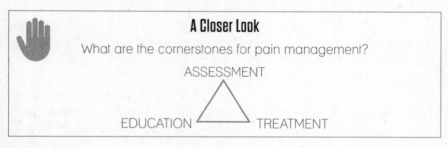

A Closer Look

What are the cornerstones for pain management?

ASSESSMENT

EDUCATION — TREATMENT

Chapter 1

State of Pain Management

The public health crisis in the United States has led to a call for change in the medical system. In the current system, the patient is defined as the one who suffers. Healthcare has been designed with disease at the center, not people. The change will require teaching people how to be healthier by integrating a variety of modalities. They will need to move away from the mentality of *fixing* to *managing* enduring diseases such as chronic pain. The current way of thinking about chronic pain management is also changing. Medical professionals and the public alike are adjusting to these new models of healthcare. Understanding more about this new approach can help improve treatment and ease the suffering related to chronic pain.

Questions for the Reader to Ponder

By the end of this chapter, you should be able to answer the following questions:

1. Does pain always mean that you are hurt and need to rest and take care of yourself until you get better?
2. Is pain part of your imagination if physicians cannot cure your pain or find out exactly what is causing it?
3. If you can lessen your pain by psychological self-control, does it mean your pain was "all in your head" to begin with?
4. Are you beyond help if you have had pain for a long time, tried everything, and nothing works?

Pain *Was* a Silent Epidemic

Until recently, pain was a silent epidemic. It is estimated that about 100 million people in the United States have chronic pain, and an additional 25 million suffer from acute pain. Approximately two-thirds of people in pain have suffered for more than five years. The most common types of pain include

- arthritis
- lower back
- bone/joint pain
- muscle pain
- fibromyalgia

We know that 36 million missed work in the last year due to pain. We also know that 83 million indicated that their pain affected participation in their activities of daily living (IOM, 2011).

A Closer Look

Do more people suffer from pain compared to other diseases?

Yes. We know that about 26 million Americans have been diagnosed with diabetes. An additional 16 million have coronary heart disease and 7 million have suffered from a stroke. Combined, these conditions add up to 23 million cases. The number of people diagnosed with cancer is about 12 million. The incidence of chronic pain is higher than heart disease, cancer, and diabetes combined! Chronic pain represents a major problem confronting our modern culture.

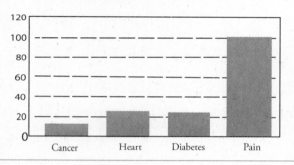

Prevalence in Millions

Pain was believed at one time to be undertreated. I have a vivid memory of watching Geraldo Rivera doing an exposé on the undertreatment of pain in nursing homes. Approximately 80% of nursing home residents who suffer from pain were found to be undertreated. About four in ten people suffered from moderate to severe pain and were unable to find adequate pain relief. We know that pain has a negative impact on an individual's quality of life and mood. Depression is the most common reaction to chronic pain, while anxiety is the most frequent reaction to acute pain.

There are also medico-legal issues that pain providers have to consider during the treatment of pain. They must provide timely and effective management of pain. They must adhere to evidence-based and consensus guidelines and policies. Some providers are excessively liberal, while others are extremely conservative in their approach to the evaluation and treatment of individuals with pain. The goal is to have providers practice in a standard way, which is why it is important for them to maintain their knowledge and skills. Providers must also be timely, accurate, and thorough in their documentation, while adhering to Health Insurance Portability and Accountability Act (HIPAA) guidelines.

It was once believed that we as human beings differed in some way in how we experienced pain. It was widely thought in the nineteenth century that racial groups varied in their physiological experiences to pain. In fact, the diagnosis of *Dysaesthesia Aethiopsis* or "an obtuse sensibility of the body" was believed to be a genetic insensitivity to pain attributed to those of African descent. In the present, minorities in the United States (African-Americans, Latinos, Asians, and so on) remain at risk for inadequate pain control. Clinical studies do report an ethnic difference in pain perception and response. There are differences within and between cultural and ethnic groups. Several factors affect how an individual identifies with their ethnic or cultural group, including

- gender
- age
- generation
- acculturation
- socioeconomic status (SES)
- ties to mother country
- primary language
- degree of isolation
- residence in ethnic neighborhoods

These factors may mediate the relationship between ethnic background and pain.

In terms of sex differences, we know that women generally report experiencing more recurrent, severe, and longer-lasting pain than men. The research also indicates that women have lower pain thresholds and tolerance to a range of pain stimuli. This is attributed to changes in sex hormones that moderate these differences. Women are more likely to participate in research studies and seek healthcare for pain than men. The research has also shown that men and women respond differently to opioid medications. However, multidisciplinary treatment produces similar treatment gains for both. There is greater female prevalence in painful conditions, such as

- dysmenorrheal pain (menstrual periods)
- labor pain
- fibromyalgia
- irritable bowel syndrome (IBS)
- temporomandibular disorder
- rheumatoid arthritis
- osteoarthritis
- migraine headaches with aura
- joint pain

Women are also more likely to experience depression and to experience more physical conditions than men.

Pain as the "5th Vital Sign"

In 1996, the American Pain Society introduced pain as the "5th vital sign." Up to that point, there were only four vital signs: pulse rate, temperature, respiration rate, and blood pressure. These vital signs indicate the state of a person's essential body functions. This 1996 initiative emphasized that pain assessment was as important as the evaluation of the other four standard vital signs. It stressed that providers need to take action when their patients report pain. The Department of Veterans Affairs (VA) recognized the value of such an approach and included it in their national pain management strategy. In 2000, the Joint Commission on Accreditation of Healthcare Organization (JCAHO) introduced standards for pain assessment and management relevant to multiple health care disciplines and settings. These standards stress the persons' rights to appropriate assessment and management of pain (JCAHO Standard RI1.2.8, 2000) and emphasized that pain should be assessed in all patients (JCAHO Standard PE1.4, 2000).

Interestingly, the quality of pain care remained unchanged between visits before and after the pain initiative. No significant changes were witnessed in subjective provider assessments, pain exams, orders to assess for pain, new analgesics, changes in existing analgesics, other pain treatments, and follow-up plans as a result of this initiative. One study looked at why this may have occurred by comparing the self-report of 79 patients to the documented report in their charts about their care. Approximately 22% had no attention to pain documented in the medical record. Another 27% had no further assessment documented in their chart. About 52% received no new therapy for pain at that visit, even though the patient reported pain had been assessed and treated. These findings highlighted that the problem lies in documentation, not in the practice of pain management. We can learn from our past mistakes, so it is important to review a brief history of pain management.

History of Pain Management

The philosophical, political, and religious meanings of pain have defined the suffering of individuals for much of history. Among the oldest known religious texts in history, we find examples of pain, such as flogging, crucifixion, and walking barefoot for miles through scorching deserts. Evidence of pain has been found in carvings on stone tablets from ancient civilizations. It was once believed that pain symptoms were manifestations of evil, magic, or demons, and that its relief only came from sorcerers, shamans, priests, or priestesses who used herbs, rites, and ceremonies as treatments. The Greeks and Romans were the first to advance the theory of sensation. The idea that the brain and the nervous system have a role in producing pain developed between the Middle Ages and the Renaissance. During the seventeenth and eighteenth centuries, the study of the body and the senses continued, and René Descartes described the first pain pathway. The sensations of pain, itchiness, nausea, and fatigue were believed to be protective.

Pain is the oldest medical problem and the universal physical affliction of mankind. Yet it has been little understood in physiology until very recently. In the nineteenth and twentieth centuries, medicine witnessed the development of anesthetics. Physician-scientists discovered that opium, morphine, codeine, and cocaine could be used to treat pain. This led to the later development of a pill found in your medicine cabinet, aspirin. Before long, anesthesia, both general and regional, was refined and applied during surgery. As the twenty-first century unfolds, advances in pain research are creating a less grim future. The future includes a better understanding of pain. We also have greatly improved treatments to maintain function and enrich quality of life.

Advances in Theory

Since the seventeenth century, there have been several different theories of pain perception. These include the Intensity, Specificity, Pattern, and Gate Control theories of pain. Intensity theory proposed that, due to the close relationship between a stimulus sensation and a reflex response, these two factors operate within identical neural circuitry by way of intensity. A stimulus, like an itch, activates neurons at a low level. A reflex response, such as soothing from scratching, generates neurons at higher levels. Evidence against Intensity theory has since developed and ultimately led into Specificity theory.

Specificity theory holds that specific pain receptors transmit signals to a "pain center" in the brain that produces the perception of pain. However, the theory does not account for the wide range of psychological factors that affect our perception of pain.

Pattern theory holds that pain signals are sent to the brain only when stimuli sum together to produce a specific pattern. Pattern theory does not suggest that the brain has any control over the perception of pain, but rather that it is a message recipient. Despite its limitations, Pattern theory did set the stage for the current philosophy, the Gate Control theory.

Ronald Melzack and Patrick Wall proposed the Gate Control Theory in 1965. The theory proposed that there is a "gate" or control system in the dorsal horn of the spinal cord. All information regarding pain carried by the nerves of the body must pass this gate before reaching the brain. When the gate is "open," the nerves can carry signals from the body to the brain, where pain is perceived. Chronic pain is believed to persistently activate this transmission to the dorsal horn through a cascade of hyperexcitable events in the nervous system, or induce it to "wind up." Over time, this phenomenon induces uncontrolled changes that lower the threshold for pain signals to be transmitted. When the gate is "closed," the nerves stop firing and no pain signal is sent to the brain. The goal of chronic pain management is to help "close" the gate.

A Closer Look

How do I open and close the gate?

There are several factors that open and close the "gate" of pain. These include physical sensations, thoughts, emotions, activity, and social factors.

Open	Close
Anger	Balance of activity
Attending to pain	Contentment
Depression/anxiety	Decreased tension
Fear	Engage in pleasurable activity
Illicit drug use	Engaging in activities
Isolation	Medications
Lack of recreation	Peace/happiness
Loneliness	Physical fitness
Muscle tension	Positive thinking
Negative thinking	Social support
Physical deconditioning	Spend time with family
Too much activity	Spend time with friends
Too much resting	View pain as controllable

An example is an adult walking into a playground. At first, the adult may feel overwhelmed by the screaming, laughing, and running around of children in the park. However, after a few minutes the adult may not notice these behaviors, yet they continue to exist. In this example, the analog of the children is the chronic pain people suffer. The pain is often "wound up," and the treatments help the person cope with and become habituated to the sensation. The treatments offered for chronic pain are able to produce this effect. They create changes in the neural pathways and synapses of the brain, a process known as neuroplasticity. The notion is that by making changes to biological, psychological, and social factors, the individual and pain provider are creating alterations to these neural processes. This then results in changes in pain perception.

The Role of the Brain in Pain

There are three general areas of the brain that are involved in pain:

1. the somatosensory cortex (responsible for sensation)
2. the frontal cortex (responsible for thinking)
3. the limbic system (responsible for emotions)

These brain regions are involved in learning and emotions and are important in the development of chronic pain. The brain uses any information it has available to interpret the pain signal. Our interpretation is a result of how these areas of the brain engage with the injury and then dictate how we perceive the pain.

The same regions of the brain that regulate pain also control our emotions. That means that emotional and physical pain are interpreted the same; the brain is unable to decipher between physical or emotional pain. Researchers have found that the same areas of the brain are responsible for processing both pain and feelings of depression. Another study showed that the part of the brain that works to diminish pain was sluggish in depressed subjects.

The brain uses many of the same chemicals responsible for regulating mood, including serotonin and norepinephrine, to transmit pain signals. Chronic pain and chronic depression both have similar effects on the nervous system as well, often intensifying perceptions of pain. It's no coincidence that many medications prescribed as antidepressants are effective in treating pain too. Medications dull physical and psychological pain (see chapter 3).

There are also rare cases of children who suffer from congenital insensitivity to pain. When these children fall down and scratch their knees, they do not cry or scream with pain. The disease deprives them of such an important natural protection as pain because their pain impulses are damaged. This is just further evidence that without the brain there is no pain. When people say "pain is all in your head," what they mean is that pain is all processed in the brain.

Definition of Pain

In 1996, the International Association for the Study of Pain (IASP) redefined pain as "an unpleasant sensory and emotional experience associated with actual or potential tissue damage, or described in terms of tissue damage, or both" (IASP, 1996). This definition is the culmination of centuries of ideas and work that have explored the concept of pain.

Types of Pain

There are several types of pain, including acute, chronic, cancer, and breakthrough pain. Acute pain has a sudden onset and lasts no more than three to six months. Acute pain resolves when the underlying cause is treated. Chronic pain persists beyond six months or the "normal" time of healing. The pain persists even if the trauma, injury, or infection resolves. Chronic pain is affected by both physical symptoms and emotional problems. Cancer pain is pain from the cancer itself as it spreads to organs, bone, or nerves. Cancer treatments can also cause pain. Breakthrough pain is shooting pain that occurs multiple times during the day without an identified cause or pattern. Breakthrough pain can occur when the person is already medicated. These types of pain can be further broken down into two types of pain, nociceptive and neuropathic pain.

Nociceptive pain is the "normal pain" that results from trauma or injury to our body's tissues. This may include surgery or an injury (sprain, scrape, burn, fracture, etc.). Examples of nociceptive pain include conditions like osteoarthritis, rheumatoid arthritis, and cancer pain. Persons with this type of pain experience it as throbbing, aching, dull, or sharp. Nociceptive pain usually fades once the injury heals or the painful stimulus is taken away.

Neuropathic pain results from damage or dysfunction of the nerves of the sensory transmission system. Examples of neuropathic pain include postherpetic neuralgia (painful shingles), diabetic neuropathy, and sciatica. Persons with this type of pain experience it as burning, tingling, or electrical shock feelings. Neuropathic pain does not always go away when the person heals or the stimulus is taken away.

Describing Pain

The numeric pain scale measures a person's pain intensity and is typically based on self-report. The numeric pain scale is an 11-point scale for adults and children over 10 years old. Scores range from 0 to 10, with "0" meaning no pain. A score from "1 to 3" means the person is in mild pain, is described as being nagging or annoying, and interferes a little with activities of daily living. A score of "4 to 6" means the person is in moderate pain and it often interferes significantly with activities of daily living. A score of "7 to 10" means they are in severe pain. When a person describes their pain as "severe," it is understood that their pain is disabling and they are unable to perform activities of daily living. A person should only report their pain as a "10" when they are in the most agonizing pain they have ever been in their entire life, which is considered an emergency and only treated in an emergency room.

At times, people who suffer from chronic pain hold unreasonable expectations about their treatment outcomes. People feel married to their pain scores. Pain scores alone have no utility. On average, a pain score of "2 to 3" is reported by people in the general population who do not suffer from chronic pain. A person who suffers from chronic pain should not expect their pain score to drop down to "0" after treatment, but reasonably closer to "2 to 3." In most people, chronic pain cannot be eliminated or cured. We must change the cure-seeking behavior. There are no quick fixes! Rather, the goal of chronic pain management should be to improve quality of life and physical functioning. Pain is the only condition in which the patient has a say about the failure of treatment. However, providers have the power to know what people want but the responsibility to give them what they need.

A Closer Look

What does my pain score mean?

A pain scale measures a person's pain intensity. Pain scales are based on trust. Self-report is considered the primary way to assess for pain in individuals. You will often see a sign similar to the one below at your provider's office to help you report your level of pain. There are several different types of scales. Some use faces or cartoons. Others may use numbers or descriptions of those numbers.

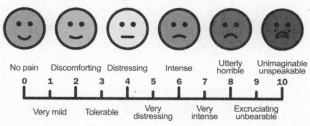

People who suffer from chronic pain can also be active contributors to their treatment. They can do this by giving more thorough information about their condition to their provider. Pain providers need detailed data to determine the causes and triggers of chronic pain in order to build a treatment plan. Unfortunately, similar language is often used to describe pain caused by different conditions, which does not assist pain providers in their assessment. Common descriptors—such as sharp, aching, throbbing, hurting, and tight—tend not to provide diagnostic distinctions between conditions. However, more unique descriptors—such as pinching, shooting, sore, and piercing—may be better labels for a lower back condition. Past research has shown that patients with systemic pain conditions, such as fibromyalgia or arthritis, describe their pain as constant, tender, tight, and cramping. Yet other pain conditions, such as migraines or headaches, may be better described as splitting, pounding, pulsating, and squeezing.

It is best if the individual is ready to provide specifics about their pain when a pain provider asks about their progress. Another way people can assist their providers is by keeping a pain diary, a consistent record of their pain experience. There have been cases where a person's description of their pain has led to a more accurate pain diagnosis, an improved treatment pain, and a better prognosis of their condition. The benefits from having additional patient information has led to task forces recommending that pain providers engage more in shared decision-making processes.

A Closer Look

What is a pain diary?

There are different examples of pain diaries available, but there are several pieces of information that are important to record. First, the provider will need to know where the pain is located. In addition, they may ask for a pain score and descriptors, which I discussed previously. Next, they will inquire about what the person with pain was doing when the pain started or increased. They will also ask whether they took any medicine, what drugs they took, and at what dosages. In addition, the provider will want to know whether the person used any other treatment to control their pain. Finally, they may ask about the results the person obtained from taking the pills, how long they took the pills, and whether there were any side effects.

Time	Where is the pain? Rate the pain (0–10) or list the word from the scale that describes your pain.	What were you doing when the pain started or increased?	Did you take medicine? What did you take? How much?	What other treatments did you use?	After an hour, what is your pain rating?	Other problems or side effects? Comments.

For Providers

Providers must also note the pain behaviors of their patients. It is normal for people to make nonverbal complaints, such as signs, gasps, moans, groans, and cries, when they are in pain. People may also make facial grimaces or wince by furrowing their brow, narrowing their eyes, clenching their teeth, tightening their lips, dropping their jaw, and distorting their expressions. People in pain will often brace themselves by clutching or holding onto furniture, equipment, or the affected area during movement. They can also become restless, constantly shifting positions, rocking, making hand motions, and being unable to keep still. They may also rub or massage the affected area and make verbal complaints, such as "ouch" or "that hurts." These behaviors are expected and are considered normal.

It is noteworthy if these behaviors are extreme, which may be an indication of illicit substance use.

What Affects Pain?

We already discussed how someone's emotional and psychological state can negatively affect their pain. If two patients with identical pain conditions present to the pain clinic and one has an untreated mental health condition, it is unclear how that person will see improvement without also addressing their mental health. In those cases, seeking professional help would be recommended in addition to their pain management.

I sometimes ask people if they would feel better if they had a free, all-expenses-paid trip to the Bahamas. When people say "yes," we discuss how their environment may be adding additional stress to them and how this affects their pain. Often, people talk about the worst pain they ever had in the past or how they are worried about their future. If someone is focused on their past, they are carrying baggage and need to address their depression. If someone is focused on the future, they are walking around worried and need to address their anxiety.

We know that some people who have pain come from families who had pain. These people may have learned behaviors during their upbringing that may be negatively affecting their pain or be in conflict with their treatment plan. Your provider needs to know what activities you are engaging in to deal with your pain other than what they have recommended.

Your expectations of and attitude toward your management can have an effect on your pain. There are two extreme examples of people who suffer from pain. You have one type who will tell you that "you don't know me or my pain" and at the same time tell you the "only thing that works is 5mg of this medication." This person is closed to suggestions and may not see any improvement in their pain. This is different from the other extreme. This person may say, "I have tried everything and nothing has worked." This person remains open to suggestions and is more likely to see improvement.

There are people with different beliefs and values, which may have an impact on their pain. For example, some religions prohibit the use of certain medical procedures due to their spiritual conflicts. It is important that your provider is aware of these beliefs. There are also social and cultural influences that may have an impact on pain. For example, there are some minorities who have a distrust of providers, which needs to be addressed before they will engage in any treatment.

I already discussed sex differences earlier, but I failed to mention age changes. We know that as we age we will slowly experience some pain. When we age, the intervertebral discs between each of our vertebrae lose their jelly and begin to flatten. When this occurs, we begin to shrink, and our internal muscular system and nervous system is compressed. This causes pain because the core of the body does not remain the same size and the internal physiology begins touching each other. So, the bad news is you may feel pain slowly as you age. This is different from the person who is 80 years old who never had pain and is now experiencing it. The new pain example is of someone who needs to be evaluated and treated.

What Does Pain Affect?

There are several areas of your life that are negatively affected by pain. We know that pain can cause stress, isolation, financial issues, and reductions in exercise and physical activity. We also know that pain changes your appetite, sleep, and mood and that it may lead some people to use illicit substances (see chapter 2). What is often not discussed is how you are addressing your pain by addressing these changes. It is a bidirectional relationship. As a caregiver or provider, if you help someone with pain address problems with their sleep or appetite (see chapter 6), they will feel better. If you help them increase their exercise (see chapter 5) or recreational activities (see chapter 6), they will become stronger and feel less pain. If you help someone address their stress levels and changes in mood (see chapter 4), this will have a positive impact on their pain. Giving or finding someone with pain social support (see chapter 8) or assistance with financial issues by helping them keep a job (see chapter 6) will relieve some of their pain. This underlines the importance of addressing all these health behaviors as part of your pain management plan.

The Pendulum Swings

Attitudes in the United States have shifted repeatedly in response to medical observations and events in legal communities. Often, providers will describe these changes as a pendulum that swings freely backward and forward. In 1961, the world had its first and only narcotic drug use conference. During that conference, there were two messages released. The first was that effective pain management was deemed a human right. The second message was to convince countries who did not allow the prescription of narcotics for pain management to use them. As you may have witnessed recently, we only get parts of the news. This led to some people believing they were entitled to opioids (what people generally call painkillers) for prolonged pain control. Providers then felt pressured to continue prescribing opioids. This reinforced their patients' beliefs and reliance on medication, which in turn reinforced bad behaviors. The role of providers is not only to reject the sole use of opioids for pain management but also to redirect people to other options and to use a multidisciplinary approach.

A Closer Look
What is chronic pain syndrome?

There are common characteristics of people who suffer from chronic pain. When someone suffers from pain for an extended period of time, this will affect their mood negatively, as previously discussed. In turn, the changes in their mood will then negatively impact their levels of activity. Often, people begin to engage more in unhealthy behaviors and less in healthy behaviors. This leads to their bodies becoming deconditioned, and the person becomes weaker. This in turn further affects their mood, which then causes the person to be unable to do things. This is a vicious cycle. The plan is to find a way for the person to get out of that cycle somehow.

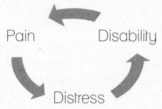

Pain — Disability — Distress

Controversy over Opioid Therapy

The use of opioids as a treatment for non-malignant chronic pain remains a subject of considerable debate. Opioids were once reserved for use in the treatment of acute and cancer pain syndromes. Nonmalignant chronic pain was considered to be unresponsive to opioids, or the use of opioids was associated with too many risks. Provider fears of regulatory pressure, medication abuse, and the development of tolerance have created a reluctance to prescribe opioids. The crossing point between legitimate medical use of opioids and its abuse and addiction continues to challenge the medical community.

There is historical evidence to suggest that opioids were related to potential harms in the past. In the sixteenth century, the first reports about addiction to opium spread throughout Europe, India, and China. By the end of the seventeenth century, there were just as many individuals addicted to morphine as there were to opium. Over the course of the eighteenth century, governments around the world began to recognize the dangers of heroin, morphine, and opium. Soon these drugs were outlawed for medicinal purposes.

In 1980, there was one study in the *New England Journal of Medicine* that found that addiction was rare in patients treated with opioids. They examined the medical files of over 11,000 patients who received at least one narcotic medication and found that there were only four cases of documented opioid addiction in patients who had a history of dependence. This study was then repeatedly referenced to justify the increase in liberal prescriptions of opioids. As of 2016, the study had been cited over 900 times in scholarly papers, according to a Google Scholar search. What these news sources failed to mention was that this study was conducted in a closed, inpatient unit where these medications were dispensed by a nurse or other provider at scheduled times. The study's findings were used to justify the release of these controlled substances to the public.

Deaths from Prescription Drug Overdose

Numerous studies of providers and specialists in pain have shown that the prescription of long-term opioids was becoming increasingly common from 1999 to 2009. Prescriptions of opioids have increased by more than 300% since 1999. The widespread dissemination of opiates coupled with lax safety measures placed on storage of these medications led to the dramatic rise of opioid misuse and deaths from overdose. In 2013, more than 16,000 people died in the United States from opioid-related overdose death (including those who died from heroin overdose). Since 2009, the leading cause of accidental death was prescription drug overdose, replacing deaths from motor vehicle accidents. The topic of opioid misuse and abuse (and the rising heroin epidemic) has dominated headlines lately. We have witnessed numerous deaths from prescription drug overdose of high profile individuals, including

- Anna N. Smith (1967–2007), model: methadone and others
- Daniel W. Smith (1986–2006), son of Anna: methadone and others
- Chris Farley (1964–1997), actor: cocaine and morphine
- Elvis Presley (1935–1977), musician: multiple drugs and codeine
- Hank Williams (1923–1953), musician: morphine and alcohol
- Heath Ledger (1979–2008), actor: multiple opiates
- Phillip S. Hoffman (1967–2014), actor: multiple drugs and opioid
- Prince (1958–2016), musician: fentanyl
- River Phoenix (1970–1993), actor: morphine and cocaine
- Sigmund Freud (1856–1939), psychoanalyst: morphine
- Tom Petty (1950–2017), musician: fentanyl and oxycodone

The United States is 5% of the world but consumes 80% of synthetic opioids created. Most other countries do not rely on these medications for pain management. People in the United States have a relationship with their medications, and they learn to become reliant on them. We are all to blame for this! This is the first man-made epidemic. It has become the #1 cause of preventable death. In 2016, the Centers for Disease Control and Prevention (CDC) finally identified this as a "public health epidemic" and released guidelines for the initiation, selection, and assessment of opioid therapy risk.

A Closer Look

Is the rate of opioid sales related to the rate of overdose deaths?

Take a look at some of the trends based on data reports below:

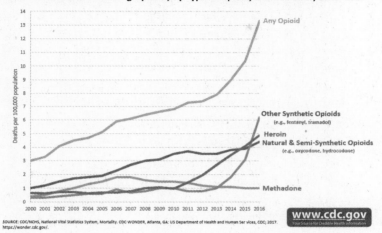

Overdose Deaths Involving Opioids, by Type of Opioid, United States, 2000-2016

SOURCE: CDC/NCHS, National Vital Statistics System, Mortality. CDC WONDER, Atlanta, GA: US Department of Health and Human Ser vices, CDC; 2017. https://wonder.cdc.gov/.

www.cdc.gov
Your Source for Credible Health Information

About 64,000 Americans died from drug overdoses in 2016, nearly double in a decade.

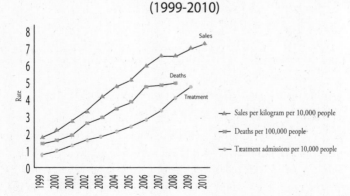

U.S. Prescription Opioid Sales, Deaths, Treatment (1999-2010)

These are according to the National Vital Statistics System (1999–2008), the Automation of Reports and Consolidated Orders System of the Drug Enforcement Administration (1999–2010), and the Treatment Episode Data Set (1999–2009).

CDC "Public Health Epidemic"

The CDC guidelines were released after several studies found that there was limited evidence supporting the benefits of long-term opioid use. The findings from these studies suggest that the risks outweigh the benefits. The CDC made 12 recommendations for prescribing opioids for chronic pain. Some are to determine when to initiate or continue opioids for chronic pain. They recommend that

1. non-opioid and non-medication strategies should be the first option for treatment for chronic pain
2. providers should assess for the risk of opioid overdose or the development of a substance use disorder during pain assessment (see chapter 2)
3. providers must be keenly aware of their patients' pain levels and their pain management strategies used when opioid medications are prescribed

Some of the recommendations are about the selection, dosage, duration, follow-up, and discontinuation of opioids. They recommend that providers

4. use immediate-release opioids when starting
5. start low and go slow
6. prescribe no more than needed when opioids are needed for acute pain and to not prescribe ER/LA opioids
7. follow up and re-evaluate risk of harm; reduce dose or taper and discontinue if needed

Some of the recommendations are for assessing risk and addressing harms of opioid use (see chapter 2 for more details). They recommend that providers

8. evaluate risk factors for opioid-related harms
9. check state prescription monitoring for high dosages and prescriptions from other providers
10. use urine drug testing to identify prescribed substances and undisclosed use
11. avoid concurrent benzodiazepine and opioid prescribing
12. arrange treatment for opioid use disorder if needed

In August 2016, the Surgeon General sent a letter to prescribers discouraging the continued prescription of opioids. Pain providers are now left with a balancing act. They are faced with balancing the needs of the person suffering from pain against the rules and regulations related to opioids and its effects on the next of kin, the community, and society at large. Providers need to remember that pain management does not equal opioids alone, and that treatment does not always equal adding something. Alexander G. Bell said:

> *"Sometimes we stare so long at a door that is closing that we see too late the one that is open."*

A Closer Look

What is the stepped care model?

There are several models available to help guide providers in pain management. In 2009, the Department of Veterans Affairs advocated for the "Stepped Care Model of Pain Management" as a best practice model. The stepped care model gives providers the ability to escalate treatment options to include specialized care and multidisciplinary approaches. Low intensity interventions requiring self-care are considered the first step, followed by a sequential process of more aggressive, expensive, and often risky interventions when appropriate. Step #2 recommends primary care assessment and management of pain conditions and can include pain health education programs. Step #3 requires a secondary consultation, including behavioral medicine and a pain clinic. Step #4 is a tertiary level of care that recommends a referral to an interdisciplinary rehabilitation facility.

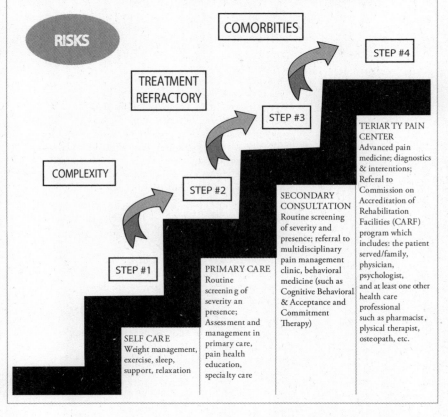

RISKS

COMORBITIES

TREATMENT REFRACTORY

COMPLEXITY

STEP #4

STEP #3

STEP #2

STEP #1

SELF CARE
Weight management, exercise, sleep, support, relaxation

PRIMARY CARE
Routine screening of severity an presence; Assessment and management in primary care, pain health education, specialty care

SECONDARY CONSULTATION
Routine screening of severity and presence; referral to multidisciplinary pain management clinic, behavioral medicine (such as Cognitive Behavioral & Acceptance and Commitment Therapy)

TERIARTY PAIN CENTER
Advanced pain medicine; diagnostics & interentions; Referal to Commission on Accreditation of Rehabilitation Facilities (CARF) program which includes: the patient served/family, physician, psychologist, and at least one other health care professional such as pharmacist, physical therapist, osteopath, etc.

Interdisciplinary/Multidisciplinary Teams

Often, the treatment of chronic pain requires the assistance of a multidisciplinary team. It is comprised of healthcare providers from several different disciplines, each addressing the pain according to their specialization. Such an approach was first employed by Dr. John Bonica during World War II and was implemented in his practice in Tacoma General Hospital. Evidence has increasingly lent support to the use of multidisciplinary pain management teams. Numerous statistical analyses and critical reviews offer clear evidence. Integrated, multidisciplinary chronic pain management programs offer people the greatest opportunity for relief of their suffering and return to functional lifestyles. These teams can range from being multidisciplinary, including two or more providers, to being interdisciplinary, which requires an interactive and cooperative interchange between a physician, a psychologist, a physical therapist, a pharmacist, and other support staff. Interdisciplinary rehabilitation programs recognize the complexities of chronic pain and require the collaborative expertise from multiple disciplines.

Discipline	Roles
Pain specialty anesthesiologists	· initial history · physical examination · review of outside records · determination of the need for diagnostic tests · detailed assessment of medication history · implementation of medication management · review findings in diagnostic tests and imaging · education of the patient · legitimize all other components of the program · interventional approaches
Physician assistant/ coordinator	· care coordinator for interdisciplinary cases · coordinate discharge plans · communicate treatment progress to providers · coordinate consults to clinic · serve as liaison between patient and staff · assist with scheduling of patients · ensure supplies are ordered and maintained · facilitate purchase of additional equipment
Psychologist	· conduct the initial psychological evaluation · implement cognitive and behavioral treatment · teach the patient coping skills · educate patients about mind-body relationship · lead patient health education programs
Registered nurses	· assess vital signs before clinic appointments · assess intervention response · act as a point of contact to coordinate care · ensure that procedures meet requirements · scrub and circulate in invasive procedures

Osteopathic physician/ physiatrist	· provide assessment · improve strength, endurance, and flexibility · help develop proper body mechanics · function mainly as teachers and coaches
Pharmacist	· patient/physician medication education · assess medication response and tolerance · co-facilitate patient health education program · provide input regarding drug interactions · track patient medication uses and dosing
Person who suffers from pain	· be considerate and respectful of everyone · discuss problems and cooperate with treatment · keep all scheduled appointments on time · provide information needed by staff · follow instructions and guidelines given · understand what medications are taken

These teams prove to be more successful when the healthcare providers involved are willing to work as a team: fostering a biopsychosocial approach, allowing the person to do the therapeutic work, and taking steps for team members to not become demoralized. The general goals of such teams are to

- identify and treat unresolved medical problems
- eliminate inappropriate medications
- improve symptoms
- restore social, occupational, and physical functioning
- restore social integration and productive employment
- reduce utilization of the health care system
- improve coping skills and foster independence

Interdisciplinary rehabilitation programs are the embodiment of the biopsychosocial model of care for people with chronic pain. Providers focus on the total person. It has long been recognized that the complexities of chronic pain require the collaborative expertise from multiple disciplines. A pain specialty physician is usually the director of the program. The patient is also considered an integral member of the team. They are responsible for self-management, which may include the use of heat/ice, stretching, walking, repositioning, and so on. The individual can make the body part feel a different way by tapping, bracing, strapping, splinting, salving, vibrating, heating, and icing.

In an ideal setting, the disciplines forming the treatment team practice at the same location. This is to maximize the common goal of improving the person's function and enhancing quality of life. According to C. Solochek of the Committee for the Accreditation of Rehabilitation Facilities, the number of accredited interdisciplinary chronic pain management programs in the United States has decreased from 210 in 1998 to only 84 in 2005. Furthermore, interdisciplinary chronic pain management programs are becoming an "endangered species" due to third-party payers, such as insurers, refusing reimbursement for treatment. They have carved out services from the interdisciplinary teams. Since access to such teams is limited and a patient's care is rarely coordinated, the need for the person to have a more active role in their pain management is emphasized. The key is for the individual and the provider to find a common ground. More recently, the term "interprofessional team" is being used to describe groups that have added Complementary & Integrative Health (see chapter 5) providers to the lineup.

Providers of these teams can also be trained as "transdisciplinary." This is a team approach to pain management that emphasizes mutual learning, training, and education, and the flexible exchange of discipline-specific roles. Providers are enabled to implement a unified, holistic, and integrated treatment plan with all members of a team responsible for the same patient-centered goals.

A Closer Look
What is a comprehensive pain management model?

By offering a multimodal approach to pain, a comprehensive pain management plan focuses on helping people to regain their life and achieve optimal outcomes. In conjunction with office visits, services may include medication management, injections/ procedures, psychological services, and other health coaching. Providers evaluate each patient and support an overall health and wellness approach. Below, you can see how different services may be recommended for different symptom reports. For example, someone who reports fatigue and inactivity may be referred to the services in the bottom right corner.

COMPREHENSIVE PAIN MANAGEMENT

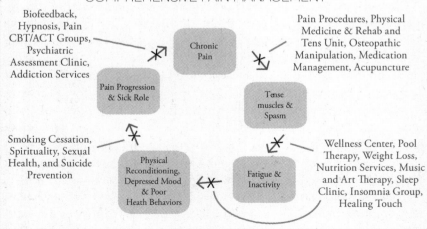

Recognized National Guidelines

The modern practice of pain management requires providers to apply evidence-based medicine to the decision-making process used in patient care. Evidence-based medicine involves the incorporation of the best available research evidence in deciding on chronic pain therapies. The creation of clinical practice guidelines to address specific clinical treatment issues has been one of the most useful and popular applications of evidence-based medicine. Specific pain conditions have guidelines set forth by national task forces. For example, the American College of Physicians and the American Pain Society have guidelines for the treatment of low back pain. Both organizations recognize the strength of approaching low back pain from an interdisciplinary rehabilitation method that includes pharmacological and interventional therapies. These organizations have also found good evidence that non-pharmacological therapies, such as cognitive-behavioral therapy (see chapter 4), progressive muscle relaxation (see chapter 4), exercise (see chapter 5), and spinal manipulation (see chapter 5), are moderately effective for chronic low back pain. In addition, they found fair evidence that acupuncture (see chapter 5), massage (see chapter 5), and yoga (see chapter 5) are effective for chronic low back pain.

The American Pain Society has also outlined strategies for the treatment of osteoarthritis/rheumatoid arthritis. First, patient education regarding the diagnosis, signs and symptoms, and treatment options is recommended. Furthermore, they recommend the use of self-care aides (see chapter 3), aerobic exercises/strengthening (see chapter 5), a TENS unit (see chapter 3), aquatic therapy, pharmacological options (see chapter 3), weight loss (see chapter 6), and intervention approaches (see chapter 3).

Several national organizations have made suggestions for the treatment of different chronic pain conditions, and all seem to include multiple modalities. For example, the National Headache Foundation set forth guidelines for the treatment of migraines/ headaches. Providers often recommend using preventive and abortive drug therapies in the treatment of migraines/ headaches. Many factors, known as triggers, may contribute to the occurrence of a migraine/headache. Possible triggers may be dietary (for example, caffeine, MSG, or yeast), lifestyle (for example, stress, inconsistent sleep, or fatigue), environmental (for example, smoke, weather, or motion), or hormonal/physical (for example, asthma medication, pregnancy, or water pills) in nature. Again, people may be able to use a pain diary to record these events and how they affect their migraines/ headaches, and then share them with their pain provider. The goal of treatment would then be for the person to avoid these identified triggers and engage in healthier lifestyle choices. Alternatively, nonpharmacological treatments, such as relaxation/biofeedback (see chapter 4), hypnosis (see chapter 4), acupuncture (see chapter 5), physical medicine (see chapter 3), and behavioral medicine such as cognitive-behavioral therapy (see chapter 4), may also provide relief.

This pattern of using multiple pain treatment modalities seems to generalize to widespread musculoskeletal pain conditions, such as fibromyalgia. Guidelines for the treatment of fibromyalgia have been proposed by the Family Nurse Practitioner Program at the School of Nursing at University of Texas. They recommend that people diagnosed with fibromyalgia and their families both receive education regarding the diagnosis, signs and symptoms, and treatment options. They also suggest treatment that includes pharmacological therapy, such as antidepressants, anticonvulsants, and other medications (such as cyclobenzaprine and tramadol). In addition, they recommend non-pharmacological interventions, including aerobic exercise/strength training, cognitive-behavioral therapy, acupuncture, hypnosis, and relaxation/biofeedback.

Need for Telemedicine

Telemedicine harnesses technology to bridge geographical distance and connects providers and chronic pain specialists as they jointly seek to help people in a more effective, holistic way. Telemedicine is the clinical application of consultative, preventative, diagnostic, and therapeutic services via two-way interactive telecommunication technology. Despite established success, it is underused for pain. There are different kinds of telemedicine, including

- telephone (such as FaceTime on the iPhone)
- internet (such as Skype)
- video conferencing
- at-home patient monitoring
- wearable technology

Sometimes, telemedicine will be used to provide a "Scan-Echo" training. These trainings use case-based presentations for providers and are often located at smaller facilities or in rural areas. They are designed to increase provider knowledge, competencies, and professional training hours in a specific specialty area. Albert Einstein said:

"It has become appallingly clear our technology has surpassed our humanity."

Today's cellular phones are like little pocket supercomputers we constantly carry around with us, supplying useful information. Below is a listing of apps by genre that you may find helpful to assist you in your pain management:

PAIN SPECIFIC
My Pain Diary: Chronic Pain
Pain Killer 2.0-Binaural Beats
Chronic Pain Tracker
PainScale Pain Diary/Coach
CatchMyPain
FibroMapp

MEDICATIONS
MedCoach
MediSafe
DoseCast
Medhelper
Pillbox

MENTAL HEALTH
Insight Timer
Lantern Health
Pacifica for Stress
PTSD/ACT/Mood Coach
Talkspace Online
Anger & Irritability Management Skills

LIFESTYLE
FitStar Yoga
Map My Run
MOVE! (Weight Loss) Coach
Stay Quit (Tobacco) Coach
EMTCP Music App
YOGAmazing
Acupressure: Heal Yourself
Fooducate

SLEEP
CBT-I Coach
Simply Noise
SleepCycle

MEDITATION/BIOFEEDBACK
Headspace
Brainwave
Mindfulness Coach
Simply Being
Breath2Relax
Pain Relief Hypnosis

Biopsychosocial Model

Traditional "biomedical" methods used to treat acute pain have proven unacceptable in the treatment of chronic, or persistent, non-cancer pain. Biomedical methods tend to utilize technology as their diagnostic strategy, are short term in time, assess the cause, and define pain as a symptom, which separates the body and mind relationship. Single modalities of treatment, whether they are medications, injections/procedures, exercises, psychotherapies, or alternative therapies, have rarely been found to be sufficient in the treatment of chronic pain. Thus, the rules about treating chronic pain have changed in the medical field in the past two decades. Government task forces in the United States have suggested that if pain persists beyond six months, or the normal time of healing, then the person should be approached using the "biopsychosocial" method.

A Closer Look
What is the biopsychosocial model?

The biopsychosocial method not only suggests that the pain provider identify biomedical factors but also encourages them to focus on the psychological and social elements of the individual that are believed to be responsible for the persistence of the pain. Biopsychosocial methods tend to utilize comprehensive psychosocial diagnostic strategies, are long term in time, assess the effects of pain, and define pain as a complex problem, which acknowledges the need to treat the whole person, mind and body.

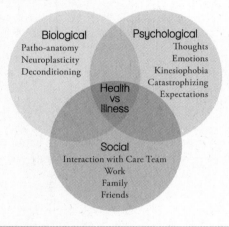

Biological
Patho-anatomy
Neuroplasticity
Deconditioning

Psychological
Thoughts
Emotions
Kinesiophobia
Catastrophizing
Expectations

Health
vs
Illness

Social
Interaction with Care Team
Work
Family
Friends

Need for Pain Education

Nelson Mandela once said:

"Education is the most powerful weapon you can use to change the world."

In 2011, the Institute of Medicine (IOM) report "Relieving Pain in America: A Blueprint for Transforming Prevention, Care, Education, and Research" was released to the public. In this report, the IOM offers a blueprint for action in transforming prevention, care, education, and research, with the goal of providing relief for people with pain in America. This report was developed because pain is a major driver for medical visits, a major reason for taking medications, a major cause of disability, and a key factor in quality of life and productivity. Given the burden of pain in human lives, dollars, and social consequences, the IOM believes that relieving pain should be a national priority. They outlined several actions that should be taken in the field of pain management:

- They suggested pain education should not be a one-time effort.
- They deemed pain management as a moral imperative.
- They outlined the value of comprehensive treatment.
- They stressed the need for interdisciplinary approaches.
- They recognized the conundrum of opioid use.
- They acknowledged the collaborative roles for patients and providers (see chapter 7).

For Providers

In terms of pain education, it is important that providers give some sort of education at every encounter. People with chronic pain have substantial unmet educational needs. At each encounter, give them a jigsaw puzzle piece, and after a few sessions they can see a full picture.

Persons with pain need to learn what is causing their pain and the rationale for therapy. They need to know why certain methods are being used for pain assessment (see chapter 2). Providers need to also set goals and realistic expectations (see chapter 7). People with chronic pain could also benefit from learning about all the treatment options available for pain management (see chapters 4 to 6). Providers need to offer education in order to change people's perspective from one of deselection (focusing on what does not work) to one of a selection of modalities.

Providers need to further educate their patients about flare-up preparation and how to assess what works. This will help to increase their confidence with education. They may also help people learn different ways to cope with pain (see chapter 8). Providers need to leave something in their patients as opposed to just giving something to them. People with pain will run through what you give them, but they can manage with what you leave in them. Ben Franklin said:

"Tell me and I forget. Teach me and I remember. Involve me and I learn."

Pain Education School Model

Some hospital systems may offer formal pain health education programs. For example, the "Pain Education School" program was developed at a Midwestern VA Medical Center on November 6, 2009, to address the health education needs of veterans who suffer from chronic, non-cancer pain. Pain Education School consists of 12 weeks of 1-hour classes with an additional 1-hour introduction class during the first week (for total of 13 hours). Classes are scheduled on a rotating basis, regardless of the patient's entry point—the providers in the study rotate on a schedule, not the patients. Over the course of the program, more than 20 interventions are presented (averaging 30 minutes each):

1. Pain Clinic (see chapter 3)/Osteopathic Manipulation (see chapter 5): Discuss injections/spinal procedures, review the multidisciplinary approach to pain management, and introduce osteopathic manipulation of the bones and tissues of the body.

2. Pharmacy (see chapter 3): Review classes of pain medications, create realistic expectations in pain management, and discuss how to refill medications.

3. Smoking Cessation/Addiction Services (see chapter 2): Describe how pain is affected by smoking tobacco, what it means to be "addicted," and how alcohol and other drugs affect pain.

4. Nutrition Services/Weight Management (see chapter 6): Describe how pain is affected by nutrition/diet, how pain is negatively affected by extra weight, and weight loss tactics.

5. Physical & Occupational Therapies (see chapter 3): Describe how pain is affected by the use of good body mechanics, how to maintain natural back curves and avoid swayback, what self-care aids are available, and movement-based exercises (for example, yoga, tai chi, or qigong).

6. Recreation Therapy/Sexual Health (see chapter 6): Describe how sexual health is affected by pain and how to cope with/manage pain with recreational activities, and review available therapies (such as gym, golf, equine, music/art, and aquatic).

7. Mental Health (see chapter 2)/Vocational Rehabilitation (see chapter 6): Describe how pain is affected by depression and anxiety and how pain is closely associated with suicide, and review different job skills and the benefits of employment.

8. Behavioral Programs (see chapter 4): Describe psychological interventions, including cognitive-behavioral therapy (CBT) and acceptance & commitment therapy (ACT), and the benefits of these approaches.

9. Hypnosis/Biofeedback (see chapter 4): Describe how hypnosis and biofeedback can help people cope with pain and what types of biofeedback are available.

10. Spirituality (see chapter 6)/Healing Touch (see chapter 5): Describe what is healing touch and how it treats pain, the biopsychosocial + spiritual model of pain, and how spirituality/faith/religion affects pain.

11. Insomnia/Sleep Disorders Clinic (see chapter 6): Describe how pain is affected by sleep disorders, provide information about continuous positive airway pressure (CPAP) treatment and sleep studies, and describe behavioral interventions to improve sleep hygiene and treat insomnia.

12. Acupuncture/Traditional Chinese Medicine (see chapter 5): Describe traditional Chinese medicine (TCM), including TCM theory and approach to diagnosis, how pain and other conditions are addressed by TCM, and different types of treatments offered in TCM.

Research findings from the first year of the program suggested that veterans who participated in the program

- moved from a contemplative to a preparation stage of change
- witnessed improvement in the experience of their pain
- exhibited an improvement in their mood

However, there was not a significant difference found in pain knowledge. In response to these findings, the research team assessed changes in pain knowledge using a different instrument and examined whether the addition of an active learning component (such as the use of an audience response system or ARS) led to greater increases in pain knowledge. Participants reported a significant difference in their

- pain beliefs
- stage of readiness to adopt a self-management approach
- depressive symptoms after completing the program

Veterans who used the ARS demonstrated greater increases in pain knowledge acquisition than those who did not. These findings provided support for the incorporation of ARS in pain education programming to facilitate active learning and to increase knowledge acquisition. Another study investigated whether veterans would report an increase in complementary and integrative health (CIH) utilization after completing the program. The findings indicated that there was a significant difference found in overall utilization of CIH after completing the program.

Another facet of program evaluation included incorporating feedback about the program. The research team assessed patients' satisfaction with the program within the initial two-year phase of implementation. Research findings suggested that patients reported

- learning "new and useful" information
- perceiving the program as "easy to understand"
- using the learned information
- recommending the program to others

A Closer Look

Is there a relationship between provider
and patient education?

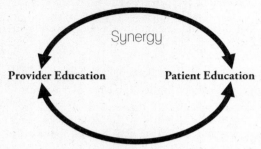

Synergy

Provider Education   **Patient Education**

We also defined and described provider satisfaction with the program. Providers found the goals and services of the program to be "clear," perceived that the strategies used "influenced" their practice, perceived that the methods of communication with the coordinators were "helpful," and perceived the program as having a "positive" impact on their service.

Additionally, providers treating patients who underwent the educational program

- received fewer complaints about pain medications
- had fewer walk-ins for pain management issues
- spent more time with their patients on other medical problems
- felt more comfortable in managing chronic pain due to the program

The results also tallied providers' level of use of the program, including the extent to which providers

- "referred patients" for this service
- never referred but used it as "a resource for assistance with chronic pain management"
- referred and used the service

Finally, the results indicated providers' perception of patient levels of fulfillment as "satisfied."

Conclusion

The current chapter introduced pain as a silent epidemic. It reviewed the advances made in policy related to the assessment and treatment of pain, including the "pain as the 5th vital sign" initiative, the history of pain management, developments in theory, and the role of the brain in pain. Pain was defined and different types of pain were outlined. You were informed on how to describe pain, what affects pain, and what does pain affect. The chapter then reviewed the current controversy over opioid therapy, including the deaths from overdoses and the CDC's reaction to these rates. The Institute of Medicine report was also reviewed, along with the recommendations for more pain education, comprehensive treatment, and interdisciplinary approaches.

References

Arnold, L., Hudson, J, Keck, P., Auchenbach, M., Javaras, K., & Hess, E. (2006). Comorbidity of fibromyalgia and psychiatric disorders. *Clinical Psychiatry*, 67 (8), 1219–25.

Ashburn, M. & Staats, P. (1999). Management of chronic pain. *The Lancet*, 353, 1865–1869.

Brown, J., Edwards, P., Atchison, J., Lafayette-Lucey, A., Wittmer, V., & Robinson, M. (2008). Defining patient-centered, multidimensional success criteria for treatment of chronic spine pain. *Pain Medicine*, 9, 851–862.

Centers for Disease Control and Prevention. (2013). Drug overdose in the United States: Fact sheet.

Chelminski PR, Ives TJ, Felix KM, et al. A primary care, multi-disciplinary disease management program for opioid-treated patients with chronic non-cancer pain and a high burden of psychiatric comorbidity. *BMC Health Serv Res*. 2005; 5(1):3.

Chou, R., Huffman, L., American Pain Society, & American College of Physicians. (2007). Non-pharmacologic therapies for acute and chronic low back pain: A review of the evidence for an American Pain Society/American College of Physicians clinical practice guideline. *Annals of Internal Medicine*, 147, 492–04.

Cosio, D., Hugo, E., Roberts, S., & Schaefer, D. (2012). A pain education school for veterans with chronic non-cancer pain: Putting prevention into VA practice. *Federal Practitioner*, 29, 23–29.

Cosio, D. & Lin, E. (2013). Effects of a pain education program for veterans with chronic, noncancer pain: A pilot study. *Journal of Pain & Palliative Care Pharmacotherapy*, 27, 340–349.

Cosio, D. & Lin, E. (2018). Overcoming the US of Passive: Increasing Active CAM Use with Pain Education. *Global Advances in Health and Medicine*.

Cosio, D. & Lin, E. (2016). Delivery of Pain Education through Picture-Telephone Videoconferencing for Veterans with Chronic, Non-cancer Pain. *Clinical & Medical Investigations Journal*, DOI: 10.15761/CMI.1000105.

Cosio, D. & Lin, E. (2015). Using Patient Pain Education to Increase Complementary & Alternative Treatment Utilization in U.S. Veterans with Chronic, Non-Cancer Pain. *Complementary Therapies in Medicine*, 23, 413–422.

DeAngelo, N. & Gordin, V. (2004). Treatment of patients with arthritis-related pain. *The Journal of the American Osteopathic Association*, 104, 2S–5S.

Dixon, K., Keefe, F., Scipio, C., Perri, L., & Abernethy, A. (2007). Psychological interventions for arthritis pain management in adults: A meta-analysis. *Health Psychology*, 26, 241–250.

Doleys DM, Olson K. (2007). *Psychological assessment and intervention in implantable pain therapies*. Minneapolis, Minn: Medtronic Inc.

Fikremariam, D. & Serafini, M. (2011). Multidisciplinary approach to pain management. Vadivelu, N. et al. (eds). *Essentials of Pain Management*, Springer Science+Business Media.

Flor, H., Fydrich, T., & Turk, D. (1992). Efficacy of multidisciplinary pain treatment centers: A meta-analytic review. *Pain*, 49, 221–230.

Gourlay D., Heit H. (2008). Pain and addiction: managing risk through comprehensive care. *Journal of Addictive Disorders*, 27, 23–30.

Gourlay D., Heit H., Almahrezi A. (2005). Universal precautions in pain medicine: A rational approach to the treatment of chronic pain. *Pain Medicine*, 6, 107–112.

Guzman, J., Esmail, R., Karjalainen, K., et al. (2001). Multidisciplinary rehabilitation for chronic low back pain: Systematic review. *British Medical Journal*, 322, 1511–1516.

Hall J, Boswell M. (2009). Ethics, law, and pain management as a patient right. *Pain Physician*, 12, 499–506.

Hubble, M., Duncan, B., & Miller, S. (1999). *The heart and soul of change: What works in therapy*. American Psychological Association.

Institute of Medicine. (IOM) (2011). Relieving Pain in America: A Blueprint for Transforming Prevention, Care, Education, and Research. Washington, DC: National Academic Press.

International Association for the Study of Pain (IASP) (1994). Part III: Pain terms, a current list with definitions and notes on usage. *Classification of Chronic Pain*. Seattle, WA.

Ives T, Chelminski P, Hammett-Stabler C, et al. (2006). Predictors of opioid misuse in patients with chronic pain: a prospective cohort study. *BMC Health Service Research*, 6, 46.1–10

Jensen, M., Johnson, L., Gertz, K., Galer, B., & Gammaitoni, A. (2013). The words patients use to describe chronic pain: implications for measuring pain quality. *Pain*, 154, 2722–2728.

Joint Commission on Accreditation of Healthcare Organizations and the National Pharmaceutical Council. (2001). *Pain: Current understanding of assessment, management, and treatments*.

Loeser, J. & Turk, D. (2001). *Bonica's management of pain (3rd edition)*, 2067–2079.

Martin, M., Scanlon, M., McCarrier, K., Wolfe, M., & Bushnell, D. (2012). How do patients with different conditions describe their pain? *ISPOR 15th Annual European Congress*, Berlin, Germany November 6th.

Moayedi, M. & Davis, K. (2013). Theories of pain: From specificity to gate control. *Journal of Neurophysiology*, 109, 5–12.

Rosenberger, P. & Kerns, R. Implementation of the VA Stepped Care Model of Pain Management. *Annals of Behavior Medicine*, 43, S265–S.

Simmons, E., Cosio, D., & Lin, E. (2015). Using audience response systems to enhance chronic, non-cancer pain knowledge acquisition among veterans. *Telemedicine & e-Health*, 21, 557–563.

Smets, E., van, Z., & Michie, S. (2007). Comparing genetic counseling with non-genetic health care interactions: Two of a kind? *Patient Education and Counseling*, 68, 225–234.

Thorne, F. & Morley, S. (2009). Prospective judgments of acceptable outcomes for pain, interference and activity: Patient-determined outcome criteria. *Pain*, 144, 262–269.

Townsend, C., Rome, J., Bruce, B., et al. (2011). Section 3-Chapter 8: Interdisciplinary pain rehabilitation programs. In Ebert & Kerns. *Behavioral and Pharmacological Pain Management*. Cambridge University Press: New York, NY.

Turk, D. (2001). Management of pain: best of times, worst of times? Clinical Journal of Pain, 17, 107-09.

Turk, D. (2006). Pain Management – Past, Present, and Future. US Neurological Disease. Website. http://www.touchneurology.com/articles/btg-pain-management-past-present-and-future?page=0,0.

University of Texas, School of Nursing, Family Nurse Practitioner Program. (2009). *Management of fibromyalgia syndrome in adults*. Austin, TX: University of Texas, School of Nursing; 1–14.

Verhaak, P., Kerssens, J., Dekker, J., Sorbi, M., & Bensing, J. (1998). Prevalence of chronic benign pain disorder among adults: A review of the literature. *Pain*, 77, 231–239.

Veterans Affairs/Department of Defense. (2010). Evidence based practice. *Management of opioid therapy (OT) for chronic pain*.

Waddell, G. (2004). *The Back Pain Revolution*. London, England: Churchill Livingstone.

Wampold, B., Mondin, G., Moody, M., et al. (1997). A meta-analysis of outcome studies comparing bona fide psychotherapies: Empiricially, "all must have prizes." *Psychological Bulletin*, 122, 203–215.

Watson, E., Cosio, D., & Lin, E. (2015). Pain Education Across VA Clinics: First study to examine provider satisfaction of a health education program catered to patients who suffer from chronic, non-cancer pain. *Practical Pain Management*, March, 50–58.

Watson, E., Cosio, D., & Lin, E. (2014). A Mixed-Methods Approach to Veteran Satisfaction with Pain Education. *Journal of Rehabilitation Research & Development*, 51(3), 503–514.

Zgierska A, Miller M, Rabago D. (2012). Patient satisfaction, prescription drug abuse, and potential unintended consequences. *JAMA*, 307, 1377–1378.

Chapter 2

Comprehensive Pain Assessments

Pain assessment is a cornerstone of pain management. The vast majority of pain practitioners recognize assessment as a valuable part of pain treatment. This is because assessment results help create a complete picture of the person per the comprehensive pain management model. Assessment results cannot precisely predict outcomes, although they can assist patients with providers to select the best treatments. I already reviewed aspects of a pain assessment in chapter 1, including words to describe pain, intensity, location, duration, and aggravating or alleviating factors. However, there is so much more information that can be gathered to help develop a treatment plan.

The current chapter will review the different types of pain assessment tools available, including a discussion of the use of psychological assessment in a pain evaluation. Common mental health disorders found in pain samples are reviewed, including depression, anxiety, personality, and substance use disorders. A focused discussion of medicinal marijuana is also included. The chapter ends with a discussion of opioids as prescription drugs and the mitigation strategies providers use to decide whether narcotics are an appropriate treatment option.

Questions for the Reader to Ponder

By the end of this chapter, you should be able to answer the following questions:

1. What aspects of health are evaluated during a comprehensive pain assessment?
2. Why should people with chronic pain seek behavioral health services?
3. What are the risk factors for suicide? What are healthy ways to cope with suicide?
4. What experiences may indicate an addiction?
5. What are the pros/cons of medicinal marijuana?

Pain Assessment Tools

There are several formal pain assessment instruments currently available and can be found with a quick online Google search. They vary in what they measure. Decisions on which to use should be based on what the provider is looking to measure. Here are a few examples of pain instruments you can use.

Pain Quality

Neuropathic Pain Questionnaire: A 12-item assessment instrument intended to measure neuropathic pain based on qualities of pain as they are inferred from pain descriptors.

A Closer Look
What is a pain body diagram?

Pain body diagrams are frequently used in clinical environments for people to describe areas of pain. The numbers of body areas of pain have previously been shown to predict disability in population-based studies.

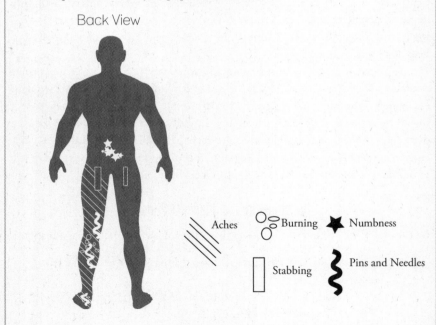

Back View

Aches   Burning   Numbness

Stabbing   Pins and Needles

Functional Impact

Brief Pain Inventory: This instrument rapidly assesses the severity of pain and its impact on functioning. It also has a pain body diagram. It has been translated into dozens of languages, and it is widely used in both research and clinical settings.

Pain Outcomes Questionnaire—VA: A 20-item inventory that functions as a multi-dimensional measure of pain in veterans to keep pace with the emergence of the biopsychosocial model of pain. It has proven to be a reliable, valid, and robust measure of the diverse cluster of symptoms associated with pain.

Sensory, Affective & Cognitive Domains

McGill Pain Questionnaire: Measures subjective pain experience and consists of 78 adjectives organized into 20 sets covering sensory, affective, and cognitive domains. People select the best descriptor in each set.

Pain Beliefs & Coping

Chronic Illness Problem Inventory: Consists of 65 self-report items related to pain behaviors, physical dysfunctions, health care behaviors, finances, sleep, relationships, and so on. It assesses coping ability, functioning, and the person's perception of problems.

Coping Strategies Questionnaire: A 50-item self-report questionnaire designed to assess 6 cognitive coping responses to pain and 2 behavioral responses.

Pain Management Inventory: An instrument that assesses specific methods that the individual is currently using for arthritis pain management and the perceived helpfulness of these methods.

Pain Self-Efficacy Questionnaire: A 10-item questionnaire developed to assess the confidence people with ongoing pain have in performing activities while in pain.

Survey of Pain Attitudes: A well-researched instrument that assesses the person's feelings about pain control, solicitous responses from others, medication, pain-related disability, pain and emotions, medical cures for pain, and pain as an indicator of physical damage or harm.

Sickness Impact Profile: A questionnaire instrument designed to measure sickness-related behavioral dysfunction and developed for use as an outcome measure in the evaluation of healthcare.

Inventory of Negative Thoughts in Response to Pain: A 12-item self-report assessment that includes three subscales: negative self-statements, negative social cognitions, and self-blame.

Level of Functioning

Oswestry Disability Questionnaire: Used to assess the person's daily functioning and activity level. Contains 10 multiple choice items that cover 9 aspects of daily living plus the use of pain medication.

Multidimensional Pain Inventory: A 52-item inventory divided into 3 sections that assess the impact of pain on the person's life, the response of significant others to the individual's communication of pain, and ability of the person to conduct common daily activities

Short-Form Health Survey: A 36-item, self-report survey of the person's health that consists of eight scaled scores, including vitality, physical functioning, bodily pain, general health perceptions, physical role functioning, emotional role functioning, social role functioning, and mental health.

Pain Disability Index: A simple and rapid instrument for measuring the impact that pain has on the ability of a person to participate in essential life activities. This can be used to evaluate the person initially, to monitor them over time, and to judge the effectiveness of interventions.

In addition to having someone in pain complete some of the instruments reviewed above, there is additional information you can note about their behavior that can help with the provider's assessment. Your assessment should begin once you meet someone. Do they call you by your first name, having never met before? How do they get up from their chair and walk toward you? Do they leave blanks on the instruments we just reviewed? All these behaviors are notable. You also may want to assess whether the person in pain has normal blood pressure. Do they have a primary care provider? Have they experienced a recent motor vehicle accident, fall, or fire, which may have worsened their pain condition? There are also more abnormal behaviors about which you should be informed, including

- multiple dose escalations of medications without medical advice
- obtaining medications from multiple sources
- selling medications
- stealing another person's medications
- forging prescriptions

A comprehensive pain assessment should include a diagnosis which differentiates between other conditions that share similar signs or symptoms and an appraisal of pain level and function. In addition, it should also include a psychological evaluation and an assessment of risk for addiction.

Psychological Assessments

Chronic pain not only affects the physical area of body but also affects mood which in turn affects behavior and then the body becomes deconditioned. We know that 1% to 3% muscle atrophy occurs per day for people lying in bed. This creates more pain, which affects emotions, and those emotions are what drive the experience of chronic pain. This creates a vicious cycle, as seen in chapter 1.

Psychology has a role to play in every aspect of pain management, including pain assessment. Behavioral health providers can help you learn ways to better manage stress or other difficult emotions connected to your pain. They can help you create a better multidisciplinary self-management plan to address your pain. In addition, they may be involved in a procedure, such as a Spinal Cord Stimulation trial, which requires a psychological evaluation. A psychological evaluation is used to assess your mental health history and may include a review of your medical file and a session in which a provider will ask questions about the following topics.

- Pain intensity/emotional pain
- What improves/negatively affects pain?
- Prior mental health treatment
- Current level of depression/anxiety
- Current use of mental health services/addiction services
- Orientation and cognitive impairment
- Suicidal ideations/homicidal ideations
- Social factors
- Substance use

A Closer Look

What is behavioral health?

Behavioral health is an umbrella term that addresses a broad range of patient issues and related healthcare services. Clinicians who have additional training in health-related conditions, medical team-based approaches, and population health management are equipped with psychological skills to address a broad array of health-related issues.

Mental Health   Diet   Substance Use
Physical Activity   Medical Conditions
Medication Management

Somatic Symptom Disorder

In psychology, chronic pain is now diagnosed as a "somatic symptom disorder" diagnosis using the Diagnostic and Statistical Manual of Mental Disorders (DSM-5). The DSM-5 updated this term from somatoform disorders. These somatic symptoms are no longer considered disordered unless they are associated with significant distress and impairment. The key change in the DSM-5 criteria is that a somatic symptom disorder diagnosis no longer requires that the somatic symptoms be medically unexplained.

Many factors contribute to a somatic symptom disorder, such as genetic/biological vulnerability (increased sensitivity to pain), early traumatic experiences (violence, abuse, and deprivation), learned behavior (experiences from prior illness that were reinforced rather than other ways of expressing distress), and cultural/social norms (which may devalue and stigmatize psychological suffering compared to physical suffering).

The new chapter of somatic symptom disorder contains several disorders, including illness anxiety (or hypochondriasis), functional neurological symptoms (or conversion disorder), factitious disorder, and psychological factors affecting other medical conditions, such as pain. These newly conceptualized diagnoses have proven more useful for primary care and medical specialists than for mental health clinicians, perhaps because patients view the reporting of somatic symptoms as a more appropriate route for seeking treatment.

Numerous studies have documented a strong association between chronic pain and mental health disorders. Previous research has shown that chronic pain is most often associated with somatoform disorders, but also depression, anxiety, personality, and substance use disorders. Thus, it is necessary to review what each of these diagnoses demands.

Depression

Depression is the fourth leading cause of disability worldwide. Investigators have found that when a pain condition is more defined, there is a lower occurrence of depression reported compared to medically unexplained pain. On the other hand, research also indicates that pain symptoms are associated with at least a two-fold increased risk for coexisting depression. In addition, it has been found that persons with multiple pain symptoms are three to five times more likely to be depressed than people without pain. The association between depression and pain also strengthens as the severity of either condition increases. Depression has been associated with a range of poor pain outcomes and worse prognosis. People with comorbid depression and pain experience more challenges in developing self-management skills.

A Closer Look

What are the actual rates that pain and mental health disorders co-occur?

In 1986, Fishbain and colleagues investigated the co-occurrence of mental health disorders in 283 chronic pain patients at the Comprehensive Pain Center of the University of Miami School of Medicine. They conducted an extensive three-day evaluation period, of which two hours were detailed, semi-structured psychiatric interviews based on the DSM-III. They found that most chronic pain patients suffer from the following:

Diagnosis	% Total
Total Anxiety	62.5
Personality	59.0
Total Depression	56.2
Substance Use	14.9
Intermittent Explosive	9.9
Dementia	7.8
Somatization	3.9
Bipolar	1.5
Obsessive-Compulsive	1.1
Psychosis	0
Sleep-wake	n/a
Dissociative	n/a

A major depressive episode is diagnosed when five or more symptoms have been present during the same two-week period nearly every day. These symptoms include

- Changes in thinking, such as difficulties thinking or concentrating and recurring thoughts of death or suicide
- Changes in feelings, such as feelings of worthlessness or guilt and depressed mood or loss of interest and pleasure (or anhedonia)
- Changes in behavior, such as significant distress or impairment in their social, occupational, or other area of functioning
- Changes in physical well-being, such as insomnia or hypersomnia, weight loss or gain, psychomotor agitation or retardation, and fatigue or loss of energy

(The depressive episode cannot be attributable to another psychological or physical condition and substance use.)

The diagnosis of major depressive disorder is based on the presence of a single or recurrent episode, current severity, psychotic features, and remission status. Depressive disorders include several other diagnoses. The common feature of these disorders is the incidence of sadness, feelings of emptiness, and/or irritability, along with somatic and cognitive changes that significantly affect the individual's function. What differs among them is their duration, timing, or presumed etiology.

Suicide Prevention

A common experience during depression and pain is to have suicidal thoughts. About 10% to 50% of people with pain have suicidal ideations. Over 30,000 suicides occur each year in this country, and it is now the 10th leading cause of death for all ages in the United States. Thus, screening for suicide among people who suffer from pain is important and can lead to a referral to a mental health professional for treatment if needed. There are several risk factors for suicide:

- Acute and chronic pain
- Sex and age
- Previous attempt/plan
- Depression, hopelessness, and other mental illness
- Substance abuse
- Medical issues
- Financial difficulty
- Rational thought loss
- Relationship problems

There are also some warning signs to look out for among people with chronic pain:

- Talking about wanting to hurt or kill themselves
- Trying to get pills, guns, or other ways to harm themselves
- Talking or writing about death, dying or suicide
- Rage, uncontrolled anger, seeking revenge
- Acting in a reckless or risky way
- Feeling trapped, like there is no way out
- Saying or feeling there's no reason for living

The most important thing to do when someone is having suicidal thoughts is to make sure they are safe. Typically, you would make sure that the person has a safety plan in place when working with someone who has suicidal thoughts. You would also make sure that they have the information to the National Suicide Hotline (1-800-273-8255). You want to encourage them to make sure to seek professional help if they are seeking mental health services with someone already. If not, you may recommend that they call 911 and have police assistance or they have someone take them to the local emergency room as a walk-in.

If the individual is not at any risk of hurting himself, I will recommend he engage in some healthy coping strategies, such as staying away from drugs and alcohol, taking a nap, taking a walk, or talking to friends. Try relaxation exercises (covered in chapter 4), distraction (covered in chapter 8), writing/reading, coloring in adult coloring books, or doing whatever works for you!

A Closer Look

Where can I find help if I have suicidal thoughts?

There are a number of resources available to help people who may be struggling with suicidal thoughts:

National Suicide Prevention Lifeline
www.suicidepreventionlifeline.org/
1-800-273-8255
Press 1 for Veterans

Here are a few other phone numbers and websites to crisis organizations:

Crisis Text Line
Text HOME to 741741

Teen Line
www.teenlineonline.org
310-855-4673

Trans Lifeline
www.translifeline.org
877-565-8860

The Trevor LGBT Project
www.thetrevorproject.org
866-488-7386

RAINN organization
www.rain.org
1-800-656-4673

Love Is Respect Project
1-866-331-9474
Text LOVEIS to 22522

It Gets Better LGBT Project
www.itgetsbetter.org

Circles of Support
www.circlesofsupport.org

Alliance of Hope for Survivors
www.allianceofhope.org

Anxiety

Anxiety disorders include conditions in which different types of objects or situations induce excessive fear, anxiety, or related behaviors. As well as feeling apprehensive and worried, you may experience some of following physical symptoms:

- Tense muscles
- Trembling
- Churning stomach/nausea/diarrhea

- Headache
- Backache
- Heart palpitations

- Numbness or "pins and needles"
- Sweating/flushing

It is easy to mistake symptoms of anxiety for physical illness and become worried that you might be suffering a heart attack or stroke. This, of course, increases anxiety.

Relative to depression, anxiety disorders have received less attention in the chronic pain literature. Anxiety disorders cause distress in more than 30 million Americans in their lifetime. The direct and indirect costs of anxiety disorders are estimated to be about $42 billion dollars per year in the United States. Anxiety disorders impair work, social life, and physical functioning.

In 2013, the American Psychiatric Association (APA), the publisher of the Diagnostic and Statistical Manual of Mental Disorders (DSM-5), decided that the chapter on anxiety disorder would no longer include post-traumatic stress disorder (PTSD). Instead, PTSD has been relocated to its own respective chapter. However, most prior research has evaluated the effects of anxiety disorders including PTSD on chronic pain and vice versa.

Post-Traumatic Stress Disorder (PTSD)

Pain is the most common physical complaint among people who suffer from PTSD. Research indicates that people with chronic pain related to trauma or PTSD experience more intense pain and affective distress, higher levels of life interference, and greater disability than their counterparts without trauma or PTSD.

DSM-5 criteria for PTSD differ significantly from those in prior editions. Criterion A is now more explicit as to whether qualifying traumatic events were experienced directly, indirectly, or witnessed by the individual; and the subjective reaction criterion was eliminated (feelings of fear, helplessness, or horror). There are also now four symptom clusters in the DSM-5:

- Re-experiencing (intrusive thoughts, nightmares, flashbacks, emotional/physiological re-experiencing)
- Alterations in arousal (irritability, aggression, self-destructive behavior, hypervigilance, exaggerated startle, problems concentrating, sleep disturbance)
- Avoidance (of external and/or internal reminders)
- Negative alterations in cognitions and mood (persistent, distorted negative beliefs, high levels of blame, strong guilt/depression/shame/horror, diminished interest, disconnection, difficulty experiencing positive emotions)

Personality Disorders

Personality traits may be described as enduring patterns of perceiving, relating to, and thinking about the environment and oneself that may be exhibited in a wide range of social and personal contexts. When these traits are inflexible, maladaptive, and lead to significant functional impairment or subjective distress, they constitute personality disorders. Research suggests that between 9% and 15% of adults in the US have at least one personality disorder, and individuals frequently present with co-occurring personality disorders from different clusters. In the chronic pain population, the rate of personality disorders ranges between 30% and 60%. Typically, personality disorders are considered to predate the onset of injury and may complicate the course of a pain syndrome. The three personality disorder clusters, all based on descriptive similarities, include

- Cluster A: Odd-eccentric, which includes paranoid, schizoid, and schizotypal personality disorders
- Cluster B: Dramatic-emotional, which includes antisocial, borderline, histrionic, and narcissistic personality disorders
- Cluster C: Anxious-fearful, which includes avoidant, dependent, and obsessive-compulsive personality disorders

Many people find it difficult to interact with individuals who suffer from a personality disorder. Each personality type requires a certain way of communicating. For example, someone who is passive, dependent, or demanding needs to be approached by the other person explaining limits in an empathic, positive, and clear manner. Here are a few other personality types and ways to behave around them.

- Someone who is dramatic, seductive, and overly affectionate may need the other person (a friend or provider) to maintain clear limits respectfully.
- Someone who is idealizing and easily disappointed may need the other person not to make promises and stop setting them up for disappointment.
- Someone who is long-suffering, masochistic, and denying may need the other person to validate their suffering.
- Someone who is orderly and controlled may need the other person to take time answering their questions or telling them they are coping the best they can.
- Someone who is somaticizing and hypochondriacal may need the other person to set up regular visits but control overuse.
- Someone who is angry, demanding, and complaining may need the other person to allow them to express their anger and offer input into decisions.

- Someone who is cold and deceitful may need the other person to avoid arguments, stop the interaction, and share reasoning when saying "no."

A Closer Look
What else should I seek help for?

It can be hard to know when you should get help. Here are some situations that might lead you to consider getting extra support:

- relationship problems
- stress from other medical problems
- stress related to trauma
- trouble managing emotional problems
- vocational issues (see more in chapter 6)

- troublesome thoughts or ideas
- confused thinking
- aggressive or self-harming behaviors
- memory problems
- homelessness
- substance abuse

Substance Use Disorders

Chronic pain is common among people being treated for substance-related disorders, and a history of substance-related disorders occurs frequently among people who receive treatment for chronic pain. However, people with chronic pain are no more likely than any other patient in the primary care setting to have a current substance use disorder, suggesting that chronic pain is not associated with unique risk for substance abuse.

The substance-related disorders are divided into two groups: substance use disorders and substance-induced disorders (such as intoxication or withdrawal). A discussion of substance-induced disorders is beyond the scope of this book. The essential feature of a substance use disorder is a cluster of cognitive, behavioral, and physical symptoms indicating that the individual continues using the substance despite significant substance-related problems. The diagnosis of a substance use disorder is based on a pathological pattern of behaviors related to use of the substance. To assist with organization, criteria can be considered to fit within four overall groupings:

- Impaired Control
  » Using more than intended or is prescribed
  » Persistent desire to use or unsuccessful attempts to quit
  » Increasing time spent using or getting
  » Craving or strong desire to use

- Social Impairment
  - » Failing to fulfill major role obligations
  - » Giving up important life activities due to use
  - » Continuing to use despite knowledge of the negative effects

- Risky Use
  - » Using in physically hazardous situations
  - » Continuing to use despite knowledge of the negative effects

- Pharmacological Criteria
  - » Tolerance, needing to use more to get the same effect
  - » Withdrawal symptoms from detoxing (nausea, insomnia, anxiety, sweating, trembling)

DSM-5 now uses a criteria count (from two to eleven) as an overall severity indicator. The number of criteria met indicates the severity, with mild (two to three criteria), moderate (four to five), and severe (six or more) disorders.

All classes of substances that are taken in excess directly activate the brain reward system. This system is involved in the reinforcement of behaviors and the production of memories. Illicit substances can produce an intense activation of that system, which then trigger the reward pathways and cause a "high" and normal activities to be neglected. Furthermore, individuals with prior lower levels of self-control may be particularly predisposed to develop substance use disorders, which may reflect impairments of brain inhibitory mechanisms. Behavioral effects of substance use disorders (repeated relapses and intense drug cravings) reflect brain changes that are evident even after detoxification when the individuals are exposed to drug-related stimuli.

Substance Use Disorder & Chronic Pain

Substance use disorder and chronic pain can be present in the same person at the same time. These two chronic diseases are said to be *comorbid*. In 2005, one study indicated that before the current opioid epidemic, approximately 32% of chronic pain patients may have had comorbid substance use disorders. In 2008, another study reported that among 5,814 patients with chronic pain who were also prescribed chronic opioid therapy, 19.5% had a current substance use disorder diagnosis documented in their medical record. Most people reported using alcohol (73%), but there were also reports of cannabis (16%), prescription and/or illicit opioids (15%), and stimulant use (cocaine 11% and amphetamines 8%). In 2011, another review found anywhere from 4% of patients with chronic pain in a primary care setting to 48% of patients with chronic pain in an AIDS clinic had a current substance use disorder. Overall, persons with a substance use disorder have been found to be at a greater risk for aberrant medication-related behaviors.

For example, if a person with a substance use disorder is prescribed an opioid, there is an increased risk for prescription opioid misuse and abuse. This is why people with comorbid substance use disorder (past and present) and chronic pain are potentially more difficult to treat and are at a higher risk for other health conditions, such as depression, anxiety, and sleep disturbances.

Substances of Abuse

The substance-related disorders encompass ten separate classes of drugs:

- alcohol
- caffeine
- cannabis
- hallucinogens (phencyclidine)
- inhalants
- opioids
- sedatives/hypnotics/anxiolytics
- stimulants (amphetamines and cocaine)
- tobacco
- other (or unknown) substances

The most commonly abused substances in people with chronic pain seems to be alcohol (current and lifetime) and narcotics (current). However, that is only when the traditional "illicit substances" are considered (not marijuana and tobacco). Each of these substances affect pain in a different way. Unfortunately, nothing works if you are using these substances.

Alcohol

People have used alcohol to relieve pain since ancient times. However, the greatest pain-reducing effects occur when alcohol is consumed at doses exceeding guidelines for moderate daily alcohol use. Withdrawal from chronic alcohol use often increases pain sensitivity, which could lead to additional drinking to reverse withdrawal-related increases in pain. Prolonged, excessive alcohol exposure can also generate painful, small-fiber peripheral neuropathies. Using alcohol with other substances to alleviate pain places people at risk for a number of harmful health consequences, including acute liver failure (with acetaminophen), gastric bleeding (with aspirin or non-steroidal anti-inflammatories), and potential overdose (with opiates).

Caffeine

Caffeine is contained in chocolate, coffee, tea, and soda. Just a single caffeinated drink stimulates your adrenal glands, the round disk-shaped organs which sit on top of each kidney in your backside. This is right in the area of the lower back. That single drink translates into the energy boost that we oftentimes seek. While this little boost is not a problem for most people on occasion, it can rapidly lead to weakened adrenals over time. Energy drinks and 5-hour shots contain large doses of caffeine and are generally discouraged. I call them "chronic pain in a bottle."

Cannabis

In 2012, cannabis was the most commonly used federally illicit drug, with more than 18 million users. More recently, the use of cannabis to address chronic pain has caused national ethical and legal discourse. When it comes to cannabis, practitioners must exercise caution when allowing their philosophical biases to influence their practice. Research with cannabis does demonstrate its efficacy in treating anorexia, vomiting from cancer chemotherapy, HIV/AIDS, and other debilitating medical disorders. There are also studies which document cannabis's therapeutic potential in pain management. However, compelling clinical trial evidence is lacking for the effectiveness of cannabis for pain management at this time.

For Providers

Providers should remain aware that there is a distinction between medicinal cannabis and recreational marijuana. Given the interplay of federal and state laws, an individual could be legally using cannabis under state law but still be in violation of federal criminal law. Thus, as a matter of federal law, providers are discouraged to prescribe cannabis or complete state medical marijuana forms. In addition, knowing the potential harms of cannabis use and its negative interactive effects with concurrent use of opioids can help guide practitioners in their clinical decision-making. Marijuana use may cause significant mental status changes, increase driving accidents, add risks in the workplace and other activities of daily living, and lead to possible substance abuse.

Hallucinogens (Phencyclidine)

The hazards of hallucinogens are mostly psychological and include panic attacks, psychotic reactions, and flashbacks. Phencyclidine, or PCP, carries a range of risks, including accidents, panic attacks, and psychotic reactions, and it is often an additive to other drugs.

Inhalants

Inhalants are an extremely popular form of substance abuse, as they are readily available and inexpensive. The most commonly abused inhalants include computer cleaner, correction fluid, lighter fluid, and glue. Inhalants may be tempting for some individuals with chronic pain, as these substances may provide physical relief, aid in sleeping, and help them cope with the effects of their condition. However, inhalant abuse is extremely dangerous and can cause instant death, lead to addiction, and cause serious health issues.

Opioids

In 2012, more than two million people used prescription drugs nonmedically for the first time in the United States. Opioid misuse can complicate pain management, and the nonmedical use of opioids has become a public epidemic. Opioid misuse can be defined as

1. a negative urine toxicological screen for prescribed opioids
2. a positive urine toxicological screen for opioids or controlled substances not prescribed by the provider
3. a positive urine toxicological screen for stimulants (cocaine or amphetamines—not prescribed by the provider)
4. evidence of procurement of opioids from multiple providers through state prescription monitoring
5. illegal distribution, including diversion of opioids and prescription forgery

People who misuse opioids may be recreational users, people with the disease of addiction, individuals who suffer from pain seeking more relief, or persons escaping emotional pain. People with nonterminal cancer should not get a free-pass because they can have the same substance use problems. About 15% of high school kids are opioid pill users. Past research has found that 29% to 60% of people with opioid addiction report chronic pain.

Sedatives/Hypnotics/Anxiolytics

Sedatives, hypnotics, and anxiolytics are often prescribed for a number of physical and psychological medical conditions. These substances reduce arousal and stimulation in various areas of the brain and cause sedation, sleep, respiratory depression, or coma. This class of substances includes all prescription sleeping medications and almost all prescription antianxiety medications. Prolonged use of these medications can be addictive for some people. These medications have also been linked to increased risk of opioid overdose, which is discussed later in this chapter.

Stimulants (Amphetamines and Cocaine)

Another medication that is often coadministered with opiates are stimulants, the third most abused prescription drug in the United States. There were more than one million nonmedical prescription drug users of stimulants identified in 2012. Stimulant prescription drugs are typically prescribed for ADHD and narcolepsy but also have a high potential for abuse. Past research has shown that prescribed amphetamines may provide an analgesic effect and enhance the analgesic effects of opioids. However, the use of prescribed stimulants with opioids has been seldom used in contemporary medicine, which may be due to their effect on blood pressure and pulse rate. Street amphetamine abuse, such as cocaine and crystal meth, comes with additional risks, including weight loss, violence, damage to organs (nasal tissue, lung function, and heart), depletion of vitamins and minerals in the body, overdose, and dependence. In 2012, nearly 2,000,000 people in America were current cocaine users, and over 400,000 people were using methamphetamine.

Tobacco

In 2012, an estimated 69 million Americans over age 12 were current users of a tobacco product. Smoking remains the leading preventable cause of premature death in the United States, with more than 20 million premature deaths since the release of the first Surgeon General's report in 1964. According to a recent study, US adults have had an estimated 14 million major medical conditions attributable to smoking. Furthermore, another recent study found that smokers were more likely to develop chronic low back pain than nonsmokers, an effect mediated by corticosteroid circuitry involved in addictive behavior and motivated learning. Medical experts say smoking can interfere with pain management and chronic pain treatment by

- causing or exacerbating painful medical conditions
- causing chronic back and neck pain by contributing to osteoporosis and deterioration of spinal discs
- contributing to joint pain found in conditions like arthritis
- increasing pain sensitivity and perception
- causing people to perceive pain more acutely
- increasing sensations and perceptions of pain
- interfering with pain medication and taking larger doses to reduce or manage pain

Other (or Unknown) Substances

There are a number of new drugs of abuse that people are using to deal with their chronic pain. Here are a few known substances:

- **Bath Salts:** Synthetic cathinones, more commonly known as "bath salts," are human-made stimulants chemically related to cathinone, a substance found in the khat plant. Human-made versions of cathinone can be much stronger than the natural product and very dangerous. Synthetic cathinones are marketed as cheap substitutes for other stimulants such as amphetamines and cocaine.
- **Flakka:** A new synthetic street drug which causes bizarre behavior, agitation, paranoia, and delusions of superhuman strength. Word on the

street is that Flakka is a combination of heroin and crack, or heroin and methamphetamines. Flakka in reality is just a newer-generation version of bath salts.

- **Kratom:** A relatively new drug to the United States that has had a ten-fold increase in use in the last few years. Kratom is the popular name for a tree; the drug comes from its leaves and has opioid-like properties. The drug may be bought in this country as a capsule filled with powdered leaf material or a chopped-up form of the leaf that can be used for tea or smoking. Most people ingest the drug.
- **Krokodil:** The medical name for the drug is desomorphine. It is made at home by acquiring codeine and cooking it with paint thinner, gasoline, hydrochloric acid, iodine, and the red phosphorus from matchsticks. The resulting liquid is injected into a vein. It is 8% to 10% more potent than morphine.
- **Loperamide:** A key ingredient in the over-the-counter diarrhea drug Imodium. There has been a ten-fold increase in reports about oral loperamide use to self-treat a discomforting opioid withdrawal or to simply get high. Sometimes called "the poor man's methadone."
- **Piperazines:** Piperazines are in a class of drug that was originally used to fight parasitic infections. They are still used as a pig wormer. Some piperazines are also used as tranquilizers. Perhaps their biggest use is recreational, and they have been nicknamed A2, Legal X, Pep X, Frenzy, or Nemesis.
- **Salvia:** An herb in the mint family found in southern Mexico. It contains opioid-like compounds that induce hallucinations. Usually, people chew fresh leaves or drink their extracted juices. The dried leaves can be smoked in rolled cigarettes, inhaled through hookahs, or vaporized and inhaled.
- **Spice:** Also known as K2. A synthetic cannabis, fake pot, synthetic marijuana, legal weed, herbal incense, and/or potpourri. Traditional smoked spice looks like herbal tobacco, but the active ingredients are synthetic cannabinoids sprayed onto the plant material.

Substance Use Treatment

Medication and psychotherapy (especially when combined) are important elements of an overall therapeutic process that often begins with detoxification, followed by treatment and relapse prevention. Naltrexone, acamprosate, and disulfiram have been FDA-approved for treating alcohol addiction; topiramate has also been showing encouraging results in clinical trials. Methadone, buprenorphine, and naltrexone are effective medications for the treatment of opiate addiction. Psychotherapy can enhance the effectiveness of medications and help people stay in treatment longer. Treatment for addiction can be delivered in many different settings using a variety of behavioral approaches. Outpatient treatment programs offer several forms of behavioral treatment, such as:

1. Cognitive-behavioral therapy, which helps people recognize, avoid, and cope with the situations in which they are most likely to abuse substances
2. Multidimensional family therapy, which addresses a range of influences on substance abuse patterns and is designed to improve overall family functioning
3. Motivational interviewing, which capitalizes on the readiness of individuals to change their behavior and enter treatment
4. Contingency management, which uses positive reinforcement to encourage abstinence from substances

Residential treatment programs are highly structured programs in which patients remain at a residence, typically for 6 to 12 months. The focus of residential treatment programs is on the resocialization of the patient to a substance-free lifestyle. A seminal 11-year, retrospective cohort study of 845 people who had been in addictions treatment found that 51% of deaths were the result of tobacco-related causes.

Tobacco Cessation

The US Preventative Services Task Force recommends that doctors ask adults 18 years of age and older about tobacco use and provide tobacco cessation interventions to those who use tobacco products. A recommended counseling strategy employs the "5-A" framework:

1. Ask about tobacco use
2. Advise to quit through clear personalized messages
3. Assess willingness to quit
4. Assist to quit
5. Arrange follow-up and support

Counseling can be brief and occur once or consist of longer or multiple sessions, with the latter being more successful. It is also more successful to combine counseling with medication than either component alone. Counseling can include developing strategies individualized to increase the chance for a successful quit attempt, including

- helping the person identify personal motivations for quitting
- monitoring smoking habits to determine smoking triggers
- creating an action plan to cope with triggers and stress
- gradual reduction of smoking

- setting a quit date
- utilizing social supports
- celebrating successes

There are many health benefits of quitting tobacco. Here is what we know:

- Within 20 minutes, your health rate and blood pressure decrease.
- Within 12 hours, the carbon monoxide level in your blood returns to normal.
- Within 3 months, your circulation and lung function improve.
- Within 9 months, you will cough less and breathe easier.
- After 1 year, your risk of coronary heart disease is cut by 50%.
- After 5 years, your risk of mouth, throat, esophagus, and bladder cancer is cut by 50%.
- After 10 years, you are half as likely to die from lung cancer.
- After 15 years, your risk of coronary heart disease is the same as a nonsmoker's.

The available FDA-approved medications for tobacco cessation include nicotine replacement therapy, sustained-release bupropion (Zyban®), and varenicline (Chantix®). Nicotine replacement therapy comes in various formulations for the person's convenience and preference, with the gum, lozenge, and transdermal patch options available without a prescription. The starting strength of the formulation is dependent on how soon the first cigarette is smoked after waking (gum and lozenge) or the total number of cigarettes smoked in a day (patch) then gradually tapered for up to 12 weeks. People should be counseled on the appropriate "chew and park" method for the nicotine replacement therapy gum to ensure proper absorption of the nicotine and to avoid food or drinks 15 minutes before or during use with either the gum or lozenge. The patch may be removed at bedtime to minimize sleep disturbances. Other formulations such as the nasal spray or oral inhaler require a prescription, with duration of therapy lasting between 3 and 6 months. Precautions with using nicotine replacement therapy formulations include recent heart attack, serious underlying cardiovascular issues, pregnancy, and breastfeeding.

The antidepressant bupropion SR (Zyban®) was the first prescription medication approved for tobacco cessation. Therapy should begin 1 to 2 weeks prior to the person's established quit date, with the duration of 7 to 12 weeks and up to 6 months in certain people. The starting dose is 150mg every morning for 3 days, and then increased to 150mg twice a day. Bupropion SR is contraindicated in people with a seizure disorder because it can lower the seizure threshold, people with a current or prior diagnosis of bulimia or anorexia nervosa, simultaneous abrupt discontinuation of alcohol or sedatives or benzodiazepines, and in individuals who have used MAO inhibitors within the past 14 days prior to therapy initiation.

Varenicline (Chantix®) is a partial nicotine agonist also approved for tobacco cessation. Therapy is initiated one week prior to the person's established quit date, with the duration of 12 weeks and up to an additional 12 weeks, if needed. The starting dose is 0.5mg every morning for the first 3 days, then increased to 0.5mg twice a day thereafter. The dose must be adjusted for severe renal impairment. Both varenicline and bupropion SR have black box warnings regarding the risk of neuropsychiatric symptoms, including changes in behavior, hostility, agitation, depressed mood, suicidal thoughts and behavior, and attempted suicide. People should be routinely monitored while on therapy and advised to contact their provider immediately if experiencing these symptoms.

A Closer Look

What other resources are available to quit smoking?

There are also national (1-877-44U-QUIT) and state tobacco quit lines (1-800-QUITNOW) as well as text messaging programs available like "smoke-freeTXT." There are several resources available to people interested in tobacco cessation:

Centers for Disease Control and Prevention Smoking & Tobacco Use
www.cdc.gov/tobacco/index.htm

American Cancer Society Guide to Quitting Smoking
www.cancer.org/healthy/stayawayfromtobacco/guidetoquittingsmoking/index

American Heart Association Quit Smoking
www.heart.org/HEARTORG/GettingHealthy/QuitSmoking/Quit-Smoking
_UCM_001085_SubHomePage.jsp

American Lung Association How to Quit Smoking
www.lung.org/stop-smoking/how-to-quit

Quit Now (U.S. Department of Health and Human Services)
betobaccofree.hhs.gov/quit-now/index.html

U.S. Department of Health and Human Services, National Institutes of Health, National Cancer Institute, USA.gov
smokefree.gov

U.S. Department of Veterans Affairs Tobacco and Health
www.publichealth.va.gov/SMOKING

Electronic cigarettes, which mimic the look and feel of regular cigarettes, are also available. They consist of a nicotine cartridge, inhaler, battery, and heating element that converts the liquid nicotine into vapor to be inhaled. Since e-cigarettes are not regulated by the FDA, manufacturers of e-cigarettes are not required to submit complete information on chemicals used, emissions, and safety. In fact, an FDA lab study in 2009 found that e-cigarettes can expose users to the same harmful chemicals found in cigarettes. The World Health Organization and the FDA do not recommend use of e-cigarettes as tobacco cessation aids, and the sales, marketing, and import have been banned in several countries.

Medicinal Marijuana

I want to start by saying that I am neither for nor against the use of medicinal marijuana. My opinion is that we are just not ready as a field to endorse the use of marijuana for chronic pain treatment. This is a political issue that has been put on the medical community to decide. I can tell you this for sure, the medical community will not recommend anyone to smoke marijuana. The lungs are not built as filter system for foreign substances but rather for the air we breathe. The medical community learned from their mistakes surrounding smoking tobacco. In addition, we do not know enough about all the components of marijuana. There are about 80 to 100 different types, about 480 components in cannabis, and 113 cannabinoids. There are three 3 classes of marijuana that are not psychologically active: CBG, CBC, and CBD. THC, CBN, CBDL, and more are classes that are psychologically active. CBD is the most abundant class and is present in 40% of resin. CBD has been shown to reduce the intensity of THC.

We do not know more about the medicinal use of marijuana because pharmaceutical companies are not getting involved. They are not conducting research into marijuana because it is schedule I and there is no federal approval for clinical trials. Marijuana is still *illegal* in the federal government. Federal law surpasses state law. As of right now, there are 29 states, plus the District of Columbia, that have legalized medicinal marijuana. CBD is still schedule I according to the DEA. There are 6 states that particularly outlaw CBD, including Idaho, South Dakota, Nebraska, Kansas, Indiana, and West Virginia. Access to medicinal marijuana varies by state, including laws about cultivation, possession, use of ID cards, diagnosis restrictions, and opened dispensaries.

Interestingly enough, there are already several different legal formulations of marijuana available in the market in the world:

- **Marinol:** A synthetic cannabinoid that can treat or prevent nausea and vomiting caused by cancer medications when other medications do not work. It can also increase the appetite of people with AIDS.
- **Nabilone:** A synthetic cannabinoid that can treat or prevent nausea and vomiting caused by cancer medications. It's used when other medications do not work.
- **Rimonabant:** An inverse agonist for the cannabinoid receptor CB1. It is an anorectic anti-obesity drug that was first approved in Europe in 2006

but was withdrawn worldwide in 2008 due to serious psychiatric side effects. It was never approved in the United States.

- **Sativex:** A specific extract of cannabis that was approved as a botanical drug in the United Kingdom in 2010 as a mouth spray to alleviate neuropathic pain, spasticity, overactive bladder, and other symptoms of MS.

There are differences between what products you buy from a pharmacy versus a dispensary. There still remain some questions regarding what you buy from a dispensary:

- **Quality control:** Has the product you are using been tested for contaminants? CBD content is real only in Colorado, Washington, Oregon, and Alaska.
- **Product form:** Which is the best route of administration—inhalation, ingestion, topical creams, vaping?
- **No warnings or reported side effects:** Adverse events among people with chronic pain include dizziness, lightheadedness, fatigue, muscle spasms, dry mouth, short-term memory impairment, suicide attempts, psychosis or mania, paranoia, agitation, motor vehicle accidents, infectious diseases, recurrent nausea and vomiting, cramping and abdominal pain, and psychological addiction.
- **No established dose to treat a condition:** In the 1970s, the THC level in marijuana was at 3.5%. Today, the THC found in marijuana averages more than 7%. Specific techniques used today can skyrocket the amount of THC to as high as 27%. Anecdotally, we suspect that marijuana helps with sleep, mood, and appetite, enhances effects of opioids, and helps offset side effects of opioids (constipation or respiratory suppression).

For Providers

If you are considering recommending the use of medicinal marijuana to someone, there are several clinical practice guidelines of which you should be aware:

- Be aware of your federal, state, institutional policies, and local laws.
- Establish goals of care for cannabis use.
- Screen for signs of misuse, abuse, and addiction.
- Counsel people on harms and risks.
- Advise on a route of administration.
- Continually monitor cannabis use, functional status, symptom severity, and use of other substances.
- Monitor other harms (motor vehicle accidents or falls).
- Advise on discontinuation or referral to substance use treatment.

Opioids as Prescription Drugs

There are many benefits to the use of opioids for the treatment of chronic pain. There is an instant attraction to opioids due to what you may have heard in the news. Some people believe it is the standard of care. People "feel something" when they take an opioid. It can also serve as an anxiolytic and can be sedating for sleep. It is available at any hospital or pharmacy no matter how remote the location. The opioid can be transported in a bottle, and the only thing you have to do is take it. Insurance companies reimburse for opioid prescriptions, and they are easy to dispense. It is easy to see how we have developed an epidemic in this country by looking at these benefits. However, there are serious risks in using opioids for the treatment of chronic pain. We know that 8% to 10% of people will get addicted to opioids. Long-term use of opioids is associated with side effects, including drowsiness, constipation, and depressed breathing. Despite the widely held perception that opioids are the most potent medications available for the treatment of pain, there is also little evidence that they are more effective than other therapies discussed in chapter 3 to chapter 6. In fact, opioids are not recommended for 90% of pain disorders!

Opioid Abuse vs. Opioid Misuse

Opioid abuse (9%) and illicit drug use (16%) have been found to be common in people with chronic pain. Many frontline providers are reluctant to prescribe an opioid for chronic pain management among people with a substance use disorder in fear of misuse, abuse, or addiction. Let me clarify these terms:

- **Misuse:** using a medication for its intended condition but not as prescribed
- **Abuse:** using a medication for something other than the intended condition
- **Addiction:** out of control use of the medication or compulsively using the medication for non-pain relief

Thus, many providers implement different justification strategies in an attempt to reduce these occurrences. Several prescribers begin treatment by working their way up the "pain analgesic ladder" before prescribing an opioid. Others attempt to identify red flags to predict these occurrences, such as

- doctor shopping
- borrowing opioids
- stealing opioids
- selling their prescriptions
- prescription forgery
- reporting lost or stolen medications
- disproportionate pain
- negative interactions with other pain providers

A Closer Look

What is a pain analgesic ladder?

The World Health Organization developed a three-step ladder for cancer pain relief in adults. If pain occurs, there should be prompt oral administration of drugs in the following order: nonopioids (aspirin and paracetamol), then mild opioids (codeine), and then strong opioids (morphine) until the patient is free of pain. However, some providers use this analgesic ladder for non-cancer pain. This is incorrect because the decision to prescribe an opioid should not be based on pain level.

World Health Organization Analgesic Ladder

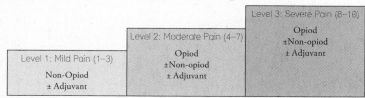

Level 1: Mild Pain (1–3)
Non-Opiod
± Adjuvant

Level 2: Moderate Pain (4–7)
Opiod
±Non-opiod
± Adjuvant

Level 3: Severe Pain (8–10)
Opiod
±Non-opiod
± Adjuvant

Taking Opioids with Benzodiazepines

The co-prescribing of benzodiazepines and opioids appears prevalent in people with substance use disorder. In fact, substance abuse treatment admissions involving the combination of benzodiazepines and opioids has increased 570% over the most recent decade. Notably, the vast majority of the 2 million nonmedical prescription drug users surveyed in 2012 were identified as nonmedical users of benzodiazepines. Most deaths from prescription drugs involved benzodiazepines (63%). Benzodiazepines are involved in 26% of opioid-related visits to the emergency room and were involved in 30% of opioid deaths.

When you add a benzodiazepine to an opioid, the risk of overdose increases tenfold. People receiving sedatives or hypnotics are also at an increased risk of opioid overdose. The co-prescribing of opioids and benzodiazepines is dangerous because of the sleep-disordered breathing associated with combined use. Both medications depress your respiration, and you can stop breathing while sleeping. An absolute contraindication of this combination of drugs includes misuse, abuse, or addiction to benzodiazepines, opioids, alcohol, or other central nervous system depressants. When both medications are present, it is recommended that you decrease and stop taking the opioid first. There is the possible risk of seizures or even death from reducing and stopping benzodiazepines first. Current research shows that when providers reduce and stop opioids, pain is reduced, function is increased, depression is reduced, and catastrophizing is reduced. Remember, decreasing and stopping medications does not mean you are getting less pain treatment!

A Closer Look

How do I know if someone's misusing or addicted?

A common concern expressed by providers is how to distinguish a person who is misusing opioids from the person who is potentially addicted. Please refer to the table below for the clinical features used to identify opioid misuse and addiction.

Clinical Features	Persons in Pain	Persons Addicted
Compulsive drug use	Rare	Common
Crave drug (when not in pain)	Rare	Common
Obtain or purchase drugs from nonmedical sources	Rare	Common
Procure drugs through illegal activities	Absent	Common
Escalate opioid dose without medical instruction	Rare	Common
Supplement with other opioid drugs	Unusual	Frequent
Demand specific opioid agents	Rare	Common
Can stop use when effective alternate treatments are available	Usually	Usually Not
Prefer specific routes of administration	No	Yes
Can regulate use according to supply	Yes	No

Naloxone Kits

Given the rapid rise of opioid overdoses, many state governments have responded by allowing local pharmacies to dispense Narcan, or naloxone, without a written prescription. This helps caregivers, concerned loved ones, first responders, and persons in pain get naloxone more easily. Naloxone is a safe and effective antidote to opioid overdoses. Naloxone works by blocking or reversing the effects of opioids. It is available as an injection or nasal spray. As of now, naloxone is available in 41 states without a prescription.

There are five steps to respond to an overdose using naloxone:

1. **Identify the overdose:** Signs of overdose are blue or pale skin color, small pupils, low blood pressure, slow heartbeat, slow or shallow breathing, snoring sound, and gasping for breath.
2. **Call 911:** Make sure to say the person is unresponsive and not breathing or struggling to breathe. Give a clear address and location. If you or the caregiver must leave, turn person on side to prevent choking on vomit.

3. **Give rescue breaths:** Giving oxygen can save someone experiencing an overdose. Perform basic CPR.
4. **Give naloxone:** If the person is still unresponsive after repeating for 30 seconds, you can give naloxone. If the person is still unresponsive in 3 to 5 minutes, you can give a second dose of naloxone.
5. **Stay until help arrives:** Stay to make sure the person doesn't go into withdrawal, take more opioids, or go back into overdose and need additional doses of naloxone.

For Providers

Mitigation Strategies

According to the new CDC guidelines for the initiation, selection, and assessment of opioid therapy risk released in March 18, 2016, providers should incorporate into the management plan strategies to mitigate risk, including an assessment and history of substance use disorder. There are several other mitigating strategies practitioners can use against opioid diversion and misuse, including

- pain management agreements
- urine toxicology screens
- opioid risk assessments
- prescription drug monitoring
- utilize universal precautions

Presently, a combination of these strategies is recommended to stratify risk, identify and understand aberrant drug related behaviors, and tailor treatments accordingly. Unfortunately, only limited data are available regarding the success of any of these strategies.

Pain Management Agreements

A pain care agreement helps people understand the provider's expectations, the short-term nature of opioid therapy, the risks that may be incurred, and the way various scenarios will be handled. For example, a pain management agreement might outline how lost or stolen opioids, requests for early refills, noncompliance with scheduled appointments, and other aberrant behaviors (diversion, doctor/pharmacy shopping, violence, and threats) will be handled. It also gives you an opportunity to discuss your specific functional goals and treatment expectations. It is recommended for everyone on chronic opioid therapy.

Urine Toxicology Screens

A urine toxicology screen should be obtained as part of the pain management agreement. It is recommended at the initial appointment and periodically while the person receives opioid therapy. The panel of substances being measured include cannabinoids, benzodiazepines, cocaine, opiates, and methadone. If a person tests positive for an illicit substance, a face-to-face discussion outlining the conditions that must be met in order to initiate or continue opioid therapy is crucial.

Opioid Risk Assessments

A risk assessment tool, such as the Screener and Opioid Assessment for Patients with Pain (SOAPP), can be used to determine the extent of monitoring required based on the person's relative risk for developing problems when placed on long-term opioid therapy. There are numerous screening tools available to help identify these individuals, including the Opioid Risk Tool, the Brief Risk Interview, the Pain Medication Questionnaire (PMQ), the Diagnosis, Intractability, Risk, Efficacy (DIRE) rating scale, the Screening Instrument for Substance Abuse Potential (SISAP), and the Drug Use Questionnaire (DAST-20).

Prescription Drug Monitoring

It may be useful to consult the prescription drug monitoring electronic database, which collects designated data on controlled substances dispensed within all 50 states. Prescription drug monitoring helps providers educate people about the use, abuse, diversion of, and addiction to prescription drugs. It helps legitimize the medical use of controlled substances for individuals. It also facilitates and encourages the treatment of prescription drug addiction. The benefit of querying your state's monitoring database is to help identify

- dangerous drug combinations
- concurrent opioid and benzo-diazepine prescriptions
- duplicative drug therapy
- other providers involved in the person's care
- patterns in person's medication compliance
- signs of aberrant behaviors and possible misuse
- multiple providers
- multiple pharmacies
- early refills

You may want to also check the prescription drug monitoring databases for your neighboring states because people are now crossing state lines to seek care for their pain management.

Other Strategies for High-Risk Cases

Providers may use random, unannounced, and witnessed sample collections. They may schedule frequent follow-up visits and/or limit the number of opioids dispensed. You may also be asked to bring in the remaining medications at your next appointment and have someone conduct a pill count.

Decision Trees for Treatment

Although there are complex guidelines for the management of opioid therapy, simplified decision support tools to guide difficult discussions and assist in determining a course of treatment for people with chronic pain are scarce. What's needed is an easy-to-use pain management "decision tree." It starts with the first step in pain management, which is identifying new or established people with a chief complaint of pain. The next step is to conduct a comprehensive pain assessment as discussed earlier. Once a decision is made to work with the person, the provider must determine whether the pain is acute or chronic and educate the individual about the difference.

For a person with chronic pain, it is helpful to outline treatment goals and consider an array of evidence-based therapies. These include non-opioid medications, physical therapy, and interventions (covered in chapter 3), and psychological interventions (covered in chapter 4). There are complementary and integrative health approaches that have been found to be successful (covered in chapter 5). This presents an opportunity to educate the person about the range of non-medication pain management strategies, attempt to integrate the person's preferences, and encourage joint decision making. It may be helpful to consider which treatment to pursue based on the intensity of pain and how invasive you wish the treatment to be. You may want to consider using a modified pain treatment ladder to determine which treatment to include in your treatment plan. It may also be helpful to expand the conversation to include treatment outcomes that focus not solely on the reduction or control of pain but on effective functioning within the context of continued pain.

Only after other treatment options have been exhausted should an opioid trial be considered. A careful risk-benefit analysis is required. Routine assessment of analgesia, activity, adverse effects, aberrant behavior, and affect will help to direct therapy. If it is determined that the risk outweighs the benefit, a referral to a pain specialist or an interdisciplinary rehabilitation program is indicated. If, on the other hand, the benefits outweigh the risks, it is crucial to ensure that the provider's practice will be able to provide adequate support. Adequate support is defined as having follow-up visits every week to month for a high-risk opioid case, and once every three months for a more stable case.

A Closer Look

What does a decision tree look like?

Decision trees are simplified decision support tools to help guide difficult discussions and assist in determining a course of treatment for people in chronic pain. This is an example of a decision tree, but trees may vary depending on the institution.

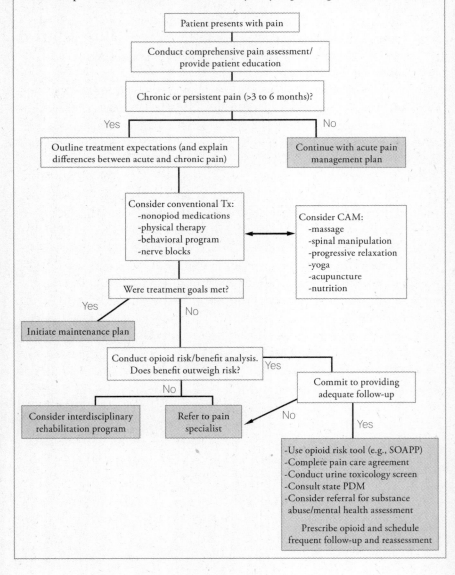

Conclusion

The current chapter reviewed the different types of pain assessment tools available. It also introduced the practice of using psychological assessment in pain evaluations. The relationships between common mental health disorders, such as depression, anxiety, personality, and substance use disorders, were explained. A focused review of the current status of medicinal marijuana was also included. I ended the chapter with a discussion of opioids as prescription drugs and the mitigation strategies providers use to decide whether narcotics are an appropriate treatment option. The next few chapters were written with the intention to provide pain education for people who suffer from chronic pain, as well as providers. I believe it is important for both to know what options are available in order to make informed decisions about the care they receive or offer.

A Closer Look

What does a modified pain ladder look like?

There are many examples of modified pain ladders available in the pain literature. I am particularly fond of using the one shown below. I use this illustration to educate people about the range of treatments available based on how invasive they are. The lowest part of the ladder shows the treatments that are the least invasive, while the upper rungs of the ladder show the more invasive.

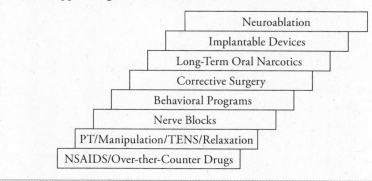

Neuroablation
Implantable Devices
Long-Term Oral Narcotics
Corrective Surgery
Behavioral Programs
Nerve Blocks
PT/Manipulation/TENS/Relaxation
NSAIDS/Over-ther-Counter Drugs

References

Amar B. (2006). Cannabinoids in medicine: A review of their therapeutic potential. *Journal of Ethnopharmacology, 105*, 1–25.

American Psychiatric Association. (1995). Practice Guideline for the Treatment of Patients with Substance Use Disorders: Alcohol, Cocaine, Opioids. *American Journal of Psychiatry, 152S*, 1–59.

American Psychiatric Association. (1996). Practice Guideline for the Treatment of Patients with Nicotine Dependence. *American Journal of Psychiatry, 153S*, 1–31.

American Psychiatric Association. (2013). *Diagnostic and statistical manual of mental disorders: DSM-5.* Washington, DC: American Psychiatric Association:

American Society of Addiction Medicine. (2001). *Patient Placement Criteria for the Treatment of Substance-Related Disorders, 2nd ed.* Chevy Chase, MD, American Society of Addiction Medicine.

Anton, R., O'Malley, S., Ciraulo, D., et al., (2006). Combined pharmacotherapies and behavioral interventions for alcohol dependence. The COMBINE study: A randomized controlled trial. *Journal of the American Medical Association, 295,* 2003–2017.

APA Society of Clinical Psychology. Borderline Personality Disorder. Available at: www.div12.org /psychologicaltreatments/disorders/borderline-personality-disorder.

Ashton C. (1999). Adverse effects of cannabis and cannabinoids. *British Journal of Anesthesiology,* 83, 637–649.

Asmundson, G., Norton, G., & Allerdings, M., et al. (1998). Post-traumatic stress disorder and work-related injury. *Journal of Anxiety Disorders,* 12, 57–69.

Atkinson, J., Slater, M., Patterson, T., et al. (1991). Prevalence, onset, and risk of psychiatric disorders in men with chronic low back pain: A controlled study. *Pain,* 45, 111–121.

Bair, M., Matthias, M., Nyland, K., et al. (2009). Barriers and facilitators to chronic pain self-management: A qualitative study of primary care patients with comorbid musculoskeletal pain and depression. *Pain Medicine,* 10, 1280–1290.

Bair, M., Robinson, R., Katon, W., & Kroenke, K. (2003). Depression and pain comorbidity: A literature review. *Archives of Internal Medicine,* 163, 2433–2445.

Ballenger, J., Davidson, J., Lecrubier, Y., et al. (2001). Consensus statement on transcultural issues in depression and anxiety from the International Consensus Group on Depression and Anxiety. *Journal of Clinical Psychiatry,* 62, 47–55.

Bao, Y., Strurm, R., & Croghan, T. (2003). A national study of the effect of chronic pain on the use of health care by depressed persons. *Psychiatric Services,* 54, 683–697.

Barry, D., Pilver, C., Potenza, M., & Desai, R. (2012). Prevalence and Psychiatric Correlates of Pain Interference Among Men and Women in the General Population. *Journal of Psychiatric Research, 46,* 118–127.

Beck, A., Emery, G., & Greenberg, R. (1985). *Anxiety Disorders and Phobias: A Cognitive Perspective.* New York: Basic Books.

Beck, A., Epstein, N., Brown, G., & Steer, R. (1988). An inventory for measuring clinical anxiety: Psychometric properties. *Journal of Consulting and Clinical Psychology,* 56, 893–897.

Beckham, J., Crawford, A., Feldman, M., et al. (1997). Chronic post-traumatic stress disorder and chronic pain in Vietnam combat veterans. *Journal of Psychosomatic Research,* 43, 379–389.

Benedikt, R. & Kolb, L. (1986). Preliminary findings on chronic pain and post-traumatic stress disorder. *American Journal of Psychiatry,* 143, 908–910.

Betrus, P., Elmore, S., & Hamilton, P. (1995). Women and somatization: Unrecognized depression. *Health Care for Women International,* 16, 287-297.

Bieling, P., Antony, M., & Swinson, R. (1998). The State-Trait Anxiety Inventory, trait version: Structure and content re-examined. *Behavior Research and Therapy,* 36, 777–788.

Blier, P. & Abbott, F. (2001). Putative mechanisms of action of antidepressant drugs in affective and anxiety disorders and pain. *Journal of Psychiatry & Neuroscience,* 26, 37–43.

Bradley L, Young L, Anderson J, et al. Effects of psychological therapy on pain behavior of rheumatoid arthritis patients: Treatment outcome and six-month follow-up. *Arthritis Rheum.* 1987; 30:1105–1114.

Breivik, H. (2005). Opioids in chronic non-cancer pain, indications and controversies. *European Journal of Pain, 9,* 127–130.

Breslau, N. & Davis, G. (1993). Migraine, physical health and psychiatric disorder: A prospective epidemiology study in young adults. *Journal of Psychiatric Research,* 27, 211–221.

Brown, R., Patterson, J., Rounds, L., & Papasouliotis, O. (1996). Substance use among patients with chronic back pain. *Journal of Family Practice, 43,* 152–160.

Burton, A., Tillotson, K., Main, C., & Hollus, S. (1995). Psychosocial predictors of outcome in acute and subchronic low back trouble. *Spine,* 20, 722–728.

Burton, K., Polatin, P., & Gatchel, R. (1997). Psychosocial factors and the rehabilitation of patients with chronic work-related upper extremity disorders. *Journal of Occupational Rehabilitation,* 7, 139–153.

Carbone, D., Schmidt, L. , Cunningham, C. , et al. (2010). Behavioral and socio-emotional functioning in children with selective mutism: A comparison with anxious and typically developing children across multiple informants. *Journal of Abnormal Child Psychology,* 38, 1057–1067.

Carroll, L., Cassidy, J., & Cote, P. (2000). The Saskatchewan Health and Back Pain Survey: the prevalence and factors associated with depressive symptomatology in Saskatchewan adults. *Canadian Journal of Public Health,* 91, 459–464.

Cavanaugh, S. (1984). Diagnosing depression in the hospitalized patient with chronic medical illness. *Journal of Clinical Psychiatry,* 45, 13–17.

Centers for Disease Control and Prevention (CDC). (2013). Web-based Injury Statistics Query and Reporting System (WISQARS) [Online]. National Center for Injury Prevention and Control, CDC. Available at: http://www.cdc.gov/injury/wisqars/index.html.

Centers for Disease Control and Prevention website. Quit Smoking Resources. Available at: http://www.cdc.gov/tobacco/quit_smoking/how_to_quit/resources/index.htm.

Chambless, D., Caputo, G., Jason, S., et al. (1985). The mobility inventory for agoraphobia. *Behavior Research and Therapy*, 23, 35–44.

Chelminski P, Ives T, Felix K, et al. (2005). A primary care, multidisciplinary disease management program for opioid-treated patients with chronic noncancer pain and a high burden of psychiatric comorbidity. *BMC Health Services Research*, 5, 3.

Chou R, Ballantyne J, Fanciullo G, et al. (2009). Research gaps on use of opioids for chronic noncancer pain: Findings from a review of the evidence for an American Pain Society and American Academy of Pain Medicine clinical practice guideline. *Journal of Pain*, 10, 147–159.

Ciechanowski, P., Katon, W., & Russo, J. (2000). Depression and diabetes: Impact of depressive symptoms on adherence, function, and costs. *Archives of Internal Medicine*, 160, 3278–3285.

Conrad R, Schilling G, Bausch C, et al. Temperament and character personality profiles and personality disorders in chronic pain patients. *Pain*. 2007;133(1-3):197–209.

Conrad R, Wegener I, Geiser F, Kleiman A. Temperament, character, and personality disorders in chronic pain. *Curr Pain Headache Rep*. 2013;17(3):318.

Cork, R., Wood, P., Ming, N., et al. (2003). The effect of cranial electrotherapy stimulation (CES) on pain associated with fibromyalgia. *The Internet Journal of Anesthesiology*, 8.

Coulehan, J., Schulberg, H., Block, M., Janosky, J., & Arena, V. (1990). Medical comorbidity of major depressive disorder in a primary medical practice. *Archives of Internal Medicine*, 150, 2363–2367.

Damush, T., Wu, J., Bair, M., Sutherland, J., & Kroenke, K. (2008). Self-management practices among primary care patients with musculoskeletal pain and depression. *Journal of Behavioral Medicine*, 31, 301–307.

Davidson, P. & Parker, K. (2001). Eye movement desensitization and reprocessing (EMDR): A meta-analysis. *Journal of Consulting and Clinical Psychology*, 69, 305–316.

Demyttenaere, I., Bruffaerts, R., Lee, S., et al. (2007). Mental disorders among persons with chronic back or neck pain: Results from the World Mental Health Surveys. *Pain*, 129, 332–342.

Department of Veterans Affairs Under Secretary for Health's Information Letter Electronic Cigarettes (E-Cigarettes), IL 10-2013-005, April 3, 2013.

Derogatis, L. (1975). Brief Symptom Inventory. Baltimore, MD: Clinical Psychometric Research.

Dersh J, Polatin PB, Gatchel RJ. Chronic pain and psychopathology: research findings and theoretical considerations. *Psychosom Med*. 2002; 64(5):773–786.

Ditre, J., Brandon, T., Zale, E., & Meagher, M. (2011). Pain, Nicotine, and Smoking: Research Findings and Mechanistic Considerations. *Psychological Bulletin, 137*, 1065–1093.

Doleys DM, Olson K. (2007). Psychological assessment and intervention in implantable pain therapies. Minneapolis, Minn: Medtronic Inc.

Elklit, A. & Christiansen, D. (2010). Acute stress disorder and PTSD in rape victims. *Journal of Interpersonal Violence*, 25, 1470–1488.

Elliott TR, Jackson WT, Layfield M, Kendall D. Personality disorders and response to outpatient treatment of chronic pain. *J Clin Psychol Med Settings*. 1996; 3(3):219–234.

Eriksen, J., Sjøgren, P., Bruera, E., Ekholm, O., & Rasmussen, N. (2006). Critical issues on opioids in chronic non-cancer pain: an epidemiological study. *Pain*, 125, 172–179.

Fabrega, H., Mezzich, J., & Mezzich, A. (1987). Adjustment disorder as a marginal or transitional illness category in DSM-III. *Archives of General Psychiatry*, 44, 567–572.

Fals-Stewart, W., O'Farrell, T., Birchler, G., et al. (2005). Behavioral couples therapy for alcoholism and drug abuse: Where we've been, where we are, and where we're going. *Journal of Cognitive Psychotherapy: An International Quarterly, 19*, 229–246.

Ferguson, R. & Ahles, T. (1998). Private body consciousness, anxiety and pain symptom reports of chronic pain patients. *Behavior Research and Therapy*, 36, 527–535.

Fink, R. (2000). Pain assessment: The cornerstone to optimal pain management. Proc (Bayl Univ Med Cent), 13, 236–239.

Fishbain, D., Cutler, R., & Rosomoff, H., & Rosomoff, R. (1998). Comorbid psychiatric disorders and chronic pain. *Current Review of Pain*, 2, 1–10.

Fishbain, D., Cutler, R., Rosomoff, H., & Rosomoff, R. (1999). Validity of self-reported drug use in chronic pain patients. *Clinical Journal of Pain*, 15, 184–191.

Fishbain, D., Goldberg, M., Meagher, B., et al. (1986). Male and female chronic pain patients categorized by DSM-III psychiatric diagnostic criteria. *Pain*, 26, 181–197.

Fleming, M., Balousek, S., Klessig, C., et al. (2007). Substance use disorders in a primary care sample receiving daily opioid therapy. *Journal of Pain*, 8, 573–582.

Gallagher, R. & Verma, S. (1999). Managing pain and comorbid depression: A public health challenge. *Seminars in Clinical Neuropsychiatry,* 4, 203–220.

Geerlings, S., Twisk, J., Beekman, A., Deeg, D., & van Tilburg, W. (2002). Longitudinal relationship between pain and depression in older adults: Sex, age, and physical disability. *Social Psychiatry and Psychiatric Epidemiology,* 37, 23–30.

Geisser, M., Roth, R., Bachman, J., & Eckert, T. (1996). The relationship between symptoms of post-traumatic stress disorder and pain, affective disturbance and disability among patients with accident and non-accident related pain. *Pain,* 66, 207–214.

Gleason, M., Fox, N., Drury, S., et al. (2011). The validity of evidence-derived criteria for reactive attachment disorder: indiscriminately social/disinhibited and emotionally withdrawn/inhibited types. *Journal of the American Academy of Child & Adolescent Psychiatry,* 50, 216–231.

Goldenberg D, et al. A controlled study of a stress-reduction, cognitive-behavioral treatment program in fibromyalgia. *J Musculoskeletal Pain.* 1994; 2:53–66.

Grant BF, Hasin DS, Stinson FS, et al. Prevalence, correlates, and disability of personality disorders in the United States: results from the national epidemiologic survey on alcohol and related conditions. *J Clin Psychiatry.* 2004; 65(7):948–958.

Grant, B., Stinson, F., Dawson, D., et al. (2004). Prevalence and co-occurrence of substance use disorders and independent mood and anxiety disorders: Results from the National Epidemiologic Survey on Alcohol and Related Conditions. *Archives of General Psychiatry,* 61, 807–816.

Greenberg, P., Sisitsky, T., Kessler, R., et al. (1999). The economic burden of anxiety disorders in the 1990s. *Journal of Clinical Psychiatry,* 60, 427–435.

Grohol, J. (2013). DSM-5 Changes: Anxiety Disorders & Phobias. Available at: https://pro.psychcentral.com/dsm-5-changes-anxiety-disorders-phobias/004266.html.

Gustin SM, Burke LA, Peck CC, Murray GM, Henderson LA. Pain and Personality: Do Individuals with Different Forms of Chronic Pain Exhibit a Mutual Personality? *Pain Pract.* 2016; 16(4):486–494.

Hah, J., Sturgeon, J., Zocca, J., et al. (2017). Factors associated with prescription opioid misuse in a cross-sectional cohort of patients with chronic non-cancer pain. *Journal of Pain Research, 10,* 979–987.

Hasin, D., O'Brien, C., Auriacombe, M., et al. (2013). DSM-5 Criteria for Substance Use Disorders: Recommendations and Rationale. *American Journal of Psychiatry, 170,* 834–851.

Herbert, J., Lilienfeld, S., Lohr, J., et al. (2000). Science and pseudoscience in the development of eye movement desensitization and reprocessing: Implications for clinical psychology. *Clinical Psychology Review,* 20, 945–971.

Hickling, E. & Blanchard, E. (1992). Post-traumatic stress disorder and motor vehicle accidents. *Journal of Anxiety Disorders,* 6, 285–291.

Hirano S, Sato T, Narita T, et al. Evaluating the state dependency of the Temperament and Character Inventory dimensions in patients with major depression: a methodological contribution. *J Affect Disord.* 2002; 69(1–3):31–38.

Hoffmann, N., Olofsson, O., Salen, B., & Wickstrom, L. (1995). Prevalence of Abuse and Dependency in Chronic Pain Patients. *International Journal of Addictions, 30,* 919–927.

Holroyd K, et al. A comparison of pharmacological and nonpharmacological therapies for chronic tension headache. *J Consult Clin Psychol.* 1991; 59:387–393.

Hurt R, Offord K, Croghan I, et al. (1996). Mortality following inpatient addictions treatment. *JAMA,* 275, 1097–1103.

Ives T, Chelminski P, Hammett-Stabler C, et al. (2006). Predictors of opioid misuse in patients with chronic pain: A prospective cohort study. *BMC Health Services Research,* 6, 46.

Jensen, M. & Patterson, D. (2006). Hypnotic treatment of chronic pain. *Journal of Behavioral Medicine,* 29, 95–124.

Jorgensen C, Boye R, Andersen D, et al. Eighteen months post-treatment naturalistic follow-up study of mentalization-based therapy and supportive group treatment of borderline personality disorder: Clinical outcomes and functioning. *Nordic Psychology.* 2014; 66(4):254–273.

Katon, W. & Schulberg, H. (1992). Epidemiology of depression in primary care. *General Hospital Psychiatry,* 14, 237–247.

Katon, W. (1984). Depression: Relationship to somatization and chronic medical illness. *Journal of Clinical Psychiatry,* 45, 4–12.

Keefe F, Caldwell D, Williams D, et al. Pain coping skills training in the management of osteoarthritic knee pain: A comparative study. *Behav Ther.* 1990; 21:49–62.

Keefe F, Gil K. Behavioral concepts in the analysis of chronic pain syndromes. *J Consul Clin Psychol.* 1986; 54:776–783.

Keefe F. Cognitive behavioral therapy for managing pain. *Clin Psychol.* 1996; 49:4–5.

Kessler, R., Chiu, W., Demler, O., et al. (2005). Prevalence, severity, and comorbidity of 12-month DSM-IV disorders in the National Comorbidity Survey Replication. *Archives of General Psychiatry,* 62, 617–627.

Kessler, R., Petukhova, M., Samson, N., et al. (2012). Twelve-month and lifetime prevalence and lifetime morbid risk of anxiety and mood disorders in the United States. *International Journal of Methods in Psychiatric Research*, 21, 169–184.

Kessler, R., Berglund, P., Demler, O. , et al. (2003). The epidemiology of major depressive disorder: Results from the National Comorbidity Survey Replication. *JAMA*, 289, 3095–3105.

Kessler, R., Ormel, J., Demler, O., & Stang, P. (2003). Comorbid mental disorders account for the role impairment of commonly occurring chronic physical disorders: Results from the National Comorbidity Survey. *Journal of Occupational & Environmental Medicine*, 45, 1257–1266.

Kinney, R., Gatchel, R., Polatin, P., et al. (1993). Prevalence of psychopadrology in acute and chronic low back pain patients. *Journal of Occupational Rehabilitation*, 3, 95–103.

Koob, G. (2006). The neurobiology of addiction: A neuroadaptational view relevant for diagnosis. *Addiction, 101S*, 23–30.

Kouyanou, K., Pither, C., Rabe-Hesketh, S., & Wessley, S. (1998). A comparative study of iatrogenesis, medication abuse, and psychiatric comorbidity in chronic pain patients with and without medically explained symptoms. *Pain*, 76, 417–426.

Kroenke, K. & Price, R. (1993). Symptoms in the community: Prevalence, classification, and psychiatric comorbidity. *Archives of Internal Medicine*, 153, 2474–2480.

Kroenke, K., Krebs, E., & Bair, M. (2009). Pharmacotherapy of chronic pain: A synthesis of recommendations from systematic reviews. *General Hospital Psychiatry*, 31, 206–219.

Lamb S, Hansen Z, Lall R, et al. Group cognitive behavioral treatment for low-back pain in primary care: A randomized controlled trial and cost-effectiveness analysis. *Lancet*. 2010; 375:916–923.

Lamb, S., Guralnik, J., Buchner, D., et al. (2000). Factors that modify the association between knee pain and mobility limitation in older women: The Women's Health and Aging Study. *Annals of Rheumatic Disorders*, 59, 331–337.

Large RG. DSM-III diagnoses of chronic pain: Confusion or clarity? *J Nerv Ment Dis*. 1986; 174(5):295–303.

Lenzenweger MF, Lane MC, Loranger AW, Kessler RC. DSM-IV personality disorders in the National Comorbidity Survey Replication. *Biol Psychiatry*. 2007; 62(6):553–564.

Mack, A. & Frances, R. (2003). Substance-related Disorders. *FOCUS: The Journal of Lifelong Learning in Psychiatry, 1*, 125–146.

Magni, G. & Merskey, H. (1987). A simple examination of the relationships between pain, organic lesions and psychiatric illness. *Pain*, 29, 295–300.

Manchikanti, L., Cash, K., Damron, K., et al. (2006). Controlled Substance Abuse and Illicit Drug Use in Chronic Pain Patients: An Evaluation of Multiple Variables. *Pain Physician, 9*, 215–226.

McFarlane, A., Atchison, M., Rafalowicz, E., & Papay, P. (1994). Physical symptoms in post-traumatic stress disorder. *Journal of Psychosomatic Research*, 42, 607–617.

McNicholas, L. (2004). *Tip 40: Guidelines for the Use of Buprenorphine in the Treatment of Opioid Addiction.* U.S. Department of Health & Human Services.

McPartland, J. & Mitchell, J. (1997). Caffeine and chronic back pain. *Archives of Physical Medicine & Rehabilitation, 78*, 61–63.

McWilliams, L., Cox, B., & Enns, M. (2003). Mood and anxiety disorders associated with chronic pain: An examination in a nationally representative sample. *Pain*, 106, 127–133.

McWilliams, L., Goodwin, R., & Cox, B. (2004). Depression and anxiety associated with three pain conditions: Results from a nationally representative sample. *Pain*, 111, 77–83.

Merikangas, K., Angst, J., & Isler, H. (1990). Migraine and psychopathology: Results of the Zurich cohort study of young adults. *Archives of General Psychiatry*, 47, 849–853.

Meyer, T., Miller, M., Metzger, R., & Borkovec, T. (1990). Development and validation of the Penn State Worry Questionnaire. *Behavior Research and Therapy*, 28, 487–495.

Michna, E., Ross, E., Hynes, W., et al. (2004). Predicting Aberrant Drug Behavior in Patients Treated for Chronic Pain: Importance of Abuse History. *Journal of Pain and Symptom Management, 28*, 250–258.

Miller, W. (1983). Motivational interviewing with problem drinkers. *Behavioral Psychotherapy, 11*, 147–172.

Miller, W. (2004). *Combined Behavioral Intervention manual: A clinical research guide for therapists treating people with alcohol abuse and dependence.* COMBINE Monograph Series, (Vol.1). Bethesda, MD: National Institute on Alcohol Abuse and Alcoholism.

Miller, W., Zweben, A., DiClemente, C., & Rychtarik, R. (1992). *Motivational Enhancement Therapy manual: A clinical research guide for therapists treating individuals with alcohol abuse and dependence.* (Volume 2, Project MATCH Monograph Series) Rockville, MD: National Institute on Alcohol Abuse and Alcoholism.

Moffitt, T., Arseneault, L., Belsky, D., et al. (2011). A gradient of childhood self-control predicts health, wealth, and public safety. *Proceedings of the National Academy of Sciences USA, 108*, 2693–2698.

Moldin, S., Scheftner, W., Rice, J., Nelson, E., Kneserich, M., & Akiskal, H. (1993). Association between major depressive disorder and physical illness. *Psychological Medicine*, 23, 755–761.

Montgomery, G., DuHamel, K., & Redd, W. (2000). A meta-analysis of hypnotically induced analgesia: How effective is hypnosis? *International Journal of Clinical & Experimental Hypnosis*, 48, 138–153.

Morasco, B., Gritzner, S., Lewis, L., et al. (2011). Systematic review of prevalence, correlates, and treatment outcomes for chronic non-cancer pain in patients with comorbid substance use disorder. *Pain*, 152, 488–497.

Morasco, B. Treatment of chronic pain in patients with comorbid substance use disorder. 2008. Available at: http://www.hsrd.research.va.gov/for_researchers/cyber_seminars/archives/563-notes.pdf.

Murray, C. & Lopez, A. (1997). Alternative projections of mortality and disability by cause 1990-2020: Global Burden of Disease Study. *Lancet*, 349, 1498–1504.

Muse, M. (1986). Stress-related, post-traumatic chronic pain syndrome: Behavioral treatment approach. *Pain*, 25, 389–394.

Najavits, L. (2009). Seeking Safety: An implementation Guide. In A Rubin and D Springer, *The Clinician's Guide to Evidence-Based Practice*. Hoboken, NJ: John Wiley.

National Center for PTSD. (2017). Clinician's Guide to Medications for PTSD. Available at: http://www.ptsd.va.gov/professional/treatment/overview/clinicians-guide-to-medications-for-ptsd.asp.

National Institute on Alcohol Abuse and Alcoholism. Using Alcohol to Relieve Your Pain: What Are the Risks? Available at: http://pubs.niaaa.nih.gov/publications/PainFactsheet/Pain_Alcohol.pdf.

National Institute on Drug Abuse. (1991). *National household survey on drug abuse: Highlights*. Washington DC: US Government Printing Office.

National Institute on Drug Abuse. (1999). *Principles of Drug Addiction Treatment: A Research-Based Guide*. NIH Pub 00-4180. Rockville, MD.

National Institute on Drug Abuse. Drug Facts: Treatment approaches for drug addiction. Available at: http://www.drug abuse.gov/publications/drugfacts/treatment-approaches-drug-addiction.

National Institutes of Health (2014). Executive summary. Pathways to prevention workshop: The role of opioids in the treatment of chronic pain. Available at: https://prevention.nih.gov/docs/ programs/p2p/ODPPainPanelStatementFinal_10-02-14 .pdf.

National Survey on Drug Use and Health (Samhsa.gov). The 10 most commonly abused drugs and their effects. Available at: https://www.duffysrehab.com/blog/top-10-most-commonly-abused-drugs-and-their-effects.

Osborn, R., Demoncada, A., & Feuerstein, M. (2006). Psychosocial interventions for depression, anxiety, and quality of life in cancer survivors: Meta-analyses. *International Journal of Psychiatry in Medicine*, 36, 13–34.

Peles, E., Schreiber, S., Gordon, J., et al. (2005). Significantly higher methadone dose for methadone maintenance treatment patients with chronic pain. *Pain*, 113, 340–346.

Perry, S., Cella, D., Falkenberg, J., et al. (1987). Pain perception in burn patients with stress disorders. *Journal of Pain and Symptom Management*, 2, 29–33.

Personality Disorder Awareness Network. Are Personality Disorders Treatable?. Available at: www.pdan.org/what-are-personality-disorders/can-pd-be-cured/#.WgMlEjYUm2w.

Pesce, A., West, C., Rosenthal, M., et al. (2010). Marijuana correlates with use of other illicit drugs in a pain patient population. *Pain Physician*, 13, 283–287.

Petre, B., Torbey, S., Griffith, J., et al. (2015). Smoking increases risk of pain chronification through shared corticostriatal circuitry. *Human Brain Mapping*, 36, 683–694.

Pitman, R., Sanders, K., Zusman, R., et al. (2002). Pilot study of secondary prevention of post-traumatic stress disorder with propranolol. *Biological Psychiatry*, 51, 189–192.

Polatin, P., Kinney, R., & Gatchel, R., et al. (1993). Psychiatric illness and chronic low-back pain. The mind and the spine—which goes first? *Spine*, 18, 66–71.

Ponte, C. & Johnson-Tribino, J. (2005). Attitudes and knowledge about pain: An assessment of West Virginia family physicians. *Family Practice*, 37, 477–480.

Potter J, Shiffman S, Weiss R. (2008). Chronic pain severity in opioid-dependent patients. *American Journal of Drug and Alcohol Abuse*, 34, 101–107.

Potter, J., Prather, K., & Weiss, R. (2008). Physical pain and associated clinical characteristics in treatment seeking patients in four substance use disorder treatment modalities. *American Journal of Addictions*, 17, 121–125.

Raphael, K., Janal, M., Nayak, S., et al. (2006). Psychiatric comorbidities in a community sample of women with fibromyalgia. *Pain*, 124, 117–125.

Regier, D., Boyd, J., Burke, J., et al. (1988). One-month prevalence of mental disorders in the United States. Based on five Epidemiologic Catchment Area sites. *Archives of General Psychiatry*, 45, 977–986.

Reisfield, G. & Webster, L. (2013). Benzodiazepines in long-term opioid therapy. *Pain Medicine*. 14, 1441–1446.

Richards A. (2015). Implications of legalized marijuana. VA Law Newsletter, 4, 2. Available at: https://vaww.ogc.vaco.portal.va.gov/Newsletter/Vol%204/Vol%204%20Issue%202%20(Spring%202015).pdf.

Rosenblum, A., Joseph, H., Fong, C., et al. (2003). Prevalence and characteristics of chronic pain among chemically dependent patients in methadone maintenance and residential treatment facilities. *Journal of the American Medical Association*, 289, 2370–2378.

Rostron, B., Chang, C., Pechacek, T. (2014). Estimation of cigarette smoking-attributable morbidity in the United States. *JAMA Internal Medicine*, 174, 1922–1928.

Sansone, R. A., Sansone, L. A. Chronic pain syndromes and borderline personality. *Innov Clin Neurosci*. 2012; 9(1):10–14.

SAVE. (2014). Suicide Facts. Suicide Awareness Voices of Education. Available at :http://www. save.org/index.cfm?fuseaction=home.viewPage&page_id=705D5DF4-055B-F1EC-3F66462866FCB4E6.

Sehgal, N., Manchikanti, L., & Smith, H. (2012). Prescription Opioid Abuse in Chronic Pain: A Review of Opioid Abuse Predictors and Strategies to Curb Opioid Abuse. *Pain Physician, 15*, ES67–ES92.

Sharp, T. (2004). The prevalence of post-traumatic stress disorder in chronic pain patients. *Current Pain and Headache Report*, 8, 111–115.

Sherman, J., Turk, D., & Okifuji, A. (2000). Prevalence and impact of post-traumatic stress disorder-like symptoms on patients with fibromyalgia syndrome. *Clinical Journal of Pain*, 16, 127–134.

Sheu, R., Lussier, D., Rosenblum, A., et al. (2008). Prevalence and characteristics of chronic pain in patients admitted to an outpatient drug and alcohol treatment program. *Pain Medicine*, 9, 911–917.

Shipherd, J., Beck, J., Hamblen, J., et al. (2003). A preliminary examination of treatment for post-traumatic stress disorder in chronic pain patients: A case study. *Journal of Traumatic Stress*, 16, 451–457.

Shipherd, J., Keyes, M., Jovanovic, T., et al. (2007). Veterans seeking treatment for post-traumatic stress disorder: What about comorbid chronic pain? *Journal of Rehabilitation Research & Development*, 44, 153–166.

Simeon, D., Hollander, E.. Treatment of personality disorders. In: *The American Psychiatric Publishing Textbook of Psychopharmacology*. Washington, DC: American Psychiatric Publishing; 2009:1267–1286.

Sonderom C, Dischinger P, Kerns T, et al. (1995). Marijuana and other drug use among automobile and motorcycle drivers treated at a trauma center. *Accident Analysis & Prevention*, 27, 131–135.

Strain, J., Smith, G. , Hammer, J., et al. (1998). Adjustment disorder: A multisite study of its utilization and interventions in the consultation-liaison psychiatric setting. *General Hospital Psychiatry*, 20, 139–149.

Surah, A., Baranidharan, G., & Morley, S. (2013). Chronic pain and depression. *Continuing Education in Anesthesia, Critical Care & Pain*, October 8th, 1–5.

Svrakic DM, Draganic S, Hill K, Bayon C, Przybeck TR, Cloninger CR. Temperament, character, and personality disorders: etiologic, diagnostic, treatment issues. *Acta Psychiatr Scand*. 2002; 106(3):189–195.

Swartz, K., Pratt, L., Armenian, H., et al. (2000). Mental disorders and the incidence of migraine headaches in a community sample: Results from the Baltimore epidemiologic catchment area follow-up study. *Archives of General Psychiatry*, 57, 945–950.

Symreng, I. & Fishman, S. (2004). Anxiety and pain. Pain Clinical Updates XII. Available at: http://iasp.files.cmsplus.com/Content/ContentFolders/Publications2/PainClinicalUpdates/Archives/PCU04-7_1390264411970_28.pdf.

Tennant F. (2011). Simultaneous use of stimulants and opioids. Practical Pain Management Online. Available at: http://www.practicalpainmanagement.com/treatments/pharmacological/opioids/simultaneous-use-stimulants-opioids.

Turk, D. & Okifuji, A. (1996). Perception of traumatic onset, compensation status, and physical findings: Impact on pain severity, emotional distress, and disability in chronic pain patients. *Journal of Behavioral Medicine*, 19, 435–453.

Turner, J., Clancy, S. Comparison of operant-behavioral and cognitive-behavioral group treatment for chronic low back pain. *J Consul Clin Psychol*. 1988; 58;573–579.

U.S. Department of Health & Human Services. (2012). *A Treatment Improvement protocol Managing Chronic Pain in Adults With or in Recovery From Substance Use Disorders: Tip 54*. Substance Abuse and Mental Health Services Administration Center for Substance Abuse Treatment Rockville, MD.

U.S. Department of Health and Human Services. Get on A Path to a Healthier You (Quitting). Available at: http://betobaccofree. hhs.gov/gallery/quit.html.

U.S. Department of Health and Human Services. The health consequences of smoking—50 years of progress: A report of the Surgeon General. Available at: http://www.surgeongeneral.gov/library/reports/50-years-of-progress/full-report.pdf.

U.S. Department of Veterans Affairs. Tobacco and Health. Available at: http://www.publichealth.va.gov/smoking/index.asp.

U.S. Preventative Services Task Force. (2009). Counseling and interventions to prevent tobacco use and tobacco-caused disease in adults and pregnant women: US Preventative Services Task Force reaffirmation recommendation statement. *Annals of Internal Medicine, 150*, 551–555.

University of California at San Francisco Rx for Change. Pharmacologic product guide: FDA-approved medications for smoking cessation. Available at: http://rxforchange.ucsf.edu/curricula/teaching_materials.php.

Van Emmerik, A., Kamphuis, J., Hulsbosch, A., & Emmelkamp, P. (2002). Single session debriefing after psychological trauma: A meta-analysis. *Lancet*, 360, 766–771.

Varni, J., Rapoff, M., Waldron, S. et al. (1996). Chronic pain and emotional distress in children and adolescents. *Journal of Developmental & Behavioral Pediatrics*, 17, 154–161.

Volkow, N. & McLellan, T. (2016). Opioid Abuse in Chronic Pain-Misconceptions and Mitigation Strategies. *New England Journal of Medicine, 374*, 1253–1263.

Von Korff, M., Dworkin, S., Le Resche, L., & Kruger, A. (1988). An epidemiologic comparison of pain complaints. *Pain*, 32, 173–183.

Watts, B., Schnurr, P., Mayo, L., et al. (2013). Meta-analysis of the efficacy of treatments for post-traumatic stress disorder. *The Journal of Clinical Psychiatry*, 74, e541–550.

Webster, L., Resifield G. (2013). Benzodiazepines in long-term opioid therapy. *Pain Medicine*, 14, 1441–1446.

Weisberg, J., Keefe, F. Personality disorders in the chronic pain population. *Pain Forum*. 1997; 6(1):1–9.

Weisberg JN. Personality and personality disorders in chronic pain. *Curr Rev Pain*. 2000; 4(1):60–70.

Wells, K., Golding, J., & Burnam, M. (1989). Affective, substance use, and anxiety disorders in persons with arthritis, diabetes, heart disease, high blood pressure, or chronic lung conditions. *General Hospital Psychiatry*, 11, 320–327.

White, P. & Faustman, W. (1989). Coexisting physical conditions among inpatients with post-traumatic stress disorder. *Military Medicine*, 154, 66–71.

Chapter 3

Traditional Approaches

In chapter 2, I reviewed how to conduct a comprehensive pain assessment, including a psychological evaluation and an assessment of addiction. The following chapters will review all of the available treatments for chronic pain. Chapter 3 introduces the traditional approaches to chronic pain management, including medications, interventions, and physical medicine and rehabilitation modalities. Most people who suffer from chronic pain are familiar with these treatment options. However, your primary care provider and/or pain medicine specialist can provide you with additional information, including the risks and benefits, about these approaches. They can also give you further information about additional traditional approaches that are not described further here.

Questions for the Reader to Ponder

By the end of this chapter, you should be able to answer the following questions:

1. What is the maximum amount of acetaminophen that should be taken in one day?
2. Which of the major side effects with opioids does not go away with chronic use?
3. Which is the lumbar area of the spine?
4. What are proper body mechanics?

Medications

Medications will always have a role in pain management. When I discuss medications, I am not only speaking of opioids or "painkillers." There are several other types of medications available for the treatment of chronic, non-cancer pain. Which medication to prescribe depends on the type, length of time, and level of your pain. Each person's response and tolerance of a pain medication is unique. Use of certain pain medications may be limited or contraindicated due to your

- other chronic conditions
- concurrent medications
- kidney or liver impairment

Therefore, medications are recommended as a part of a multidisciplinary approach to chronic pain management. Medications require constant re-evaluation regarding the risk and benefit for continuation of use. People who suffer from chronic pain should be advised

- about having realistic expectations regarding potential pain relief
- about possible side effects
- about the expected duration of therapy
- about plans for discontinuation due to intolerable side effects
- about plans for discontinuation due to lack of adequate response
- about concerns for aberrant behaviors when applicable

Medications used for chronic, non-cancer pain are classified as

- non-opioids
- opioids
- adjuvants
- steroids
- topical analgesics
- muscle relaxants

Non-Opioids

Non-opioids include acetaminophen, aspirin, and non-steroidal anti-inflammatory medications (NSAIDs). They are indicated for the treatment of mild to moderate nociceptive pain. Acetaminophen and NSAIDs are recommended for acute and chronic low back pain with self-care and non-medication therapies. Acetaminophen is available both over-the-counter (OTC) or as a prescription in combination with opioids. People who are prescribed acetaminophen should be instructed not to exceed the maximum recommended daily dose. The daily dose is limited to 3000mg/day due to risk of liver toxicity. Lower maximum doses (2000mg/day) are recommended for people with chronic liver disease or who drink alcohol. It is important for people to keep track of the total daily amount taken since many OTC products contain acetaminophen.

Unlike acetaminophen, both aspirin and NSAIDs have anti-inflammatory properties. They are used widely for arthritis, low back pain, and other musculoskeletal disorders. Aspirin and some NSAIDs are available OTC, but a majority of NSAIDs require a prescription. NSAID use should be limited to the lowest dose and shortest duration due to the risk of

- damage to the heart
- kidney toxicity
- distress to the stomach, ulcers, and bleeding

Up to 25% of chronic NSAID users will develop ulcers and 2% to 4% will bleed. There are strategies to decrease risk to the stomach, including the prescription of a proton-pump inhibitor, misoprostol, or celecoxib. People on antiplatelet therapy, like low-dose aspirin for cardio-protection, should consult their doctor prior to initiating an NSAID. Chronic NSAID use can diminish aspirin's cardio-protective effects, which can increase the risk of damage to the heart. Your doctor should evaluate your risk to the heart and stomach prior to initiating an NSAID for chronic pain management.

Opioids

Opioids are limited to the treatment of moderate to severe chronic pain. They should be considered *only* after trying all the other non-opioid and non-medication therapies. The potential benefits of prescribing an opioid must outweigh the risks. Opioids bind to receptors in the brain and spinal cord to block pain signals from the outer edge of the body. This changes the person's perception of pain. Opioids are schedule II to III controlled substances due to their risk for psychological and physical dependence. Opioids are available as short-acting, either alone or in combination with non-opioids, or as long-acting. Unlike the non-opioids that have a maximum daily dose, opioids do not have a limit. The dose is limited by associated side effects, including

- sedation
- cognitive impairment
- depression of breathing
- constipation, nausea, and vomiting

People may tolerate these side effects over time, except for constipation, which will occur throughout the duration of therapy. It is important for people on chronic opioid therapy to have a healthy bowel regimen by using a laxative with or without a stool softener. This will minimize constipation and prevent blockage. Avoid bulk-forming laxatives like psyllium, which can cause fecal loading. Sometimes people who suffer from low back pain and take opioids will see relief after having a healthy bowel movement. Remember, the colon sits towards the lower back and may be straining that area if your stool remains there.

Opioids have been shown to decrease pain scores in patients with osteoarthritis, neuropathic pain, and chronic low back pain. The majority of available studies were short in duration and used doses up to 180mg morphine equivalents per day. The results were mixed regarding the impact of opioids on patient function. Chronic opioid therapy is associated with long-term side effects including lower testosterone, low sex drive, and infertility. I find that reminding people, especially men, about this will help deter them from continued use of opioids. Other long-term side effects include

- suppressed immune system
- risk of falls and fractures in the elderly
- risk of chaotic heartbeats with use of methadone
- worsening or development of sleep apnea

- abnormal pain sensitivity leading to hyperalgesia
- risk of addiction

You may want to refer to the table below on the concept of "hyperalgesia."

Chronic opioid therapy has contributed to increases in emergency room visits, hospitalizations, and deaths from accidental overdose. The risk of accidental overdose and death increases with higher doses of opioid therapy and in combination with other sedating medications. Use of chronic opioid therapy long-term is controversial given the lack of evidence for long-term success.

A Closer Look

What is hyperalgesia?

Hyperalgesia is a contradictory response. It is when a patient taking opioids for pain actually becomes more sensitive to painful stimuli. This may be due to taking too many opioids or over-treating the pain. I tend to use an example of a two-tier chocolate cake here to help explain this concept to people. Imagine that the bottom tier of the cake is when you are prescribed a low dose of opioids. This dose has not yet reached the therapeutic dose. The thin layer of chocolate icing between the layers is the therapeutic dose. The top layer is when you are prescribed too high of a dose of opioids. When your doctor is starting an opioid trial, it is important that you follow their instructions. The doctor is trying to figure out at what point you are at the therapeutic dose. This is why it is important that you *not* experiment with your medication dosages during the trial.

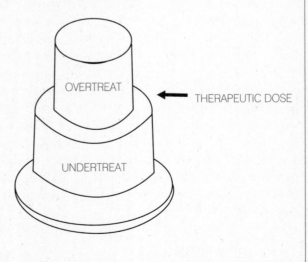

Guidelines for opioid trials recommend that your doctor review and obtain an informed consent with you that outlines

- treatment expectations
- goals of therapy as established by you
- potential risks of chronic opioid therapy
- alternatives
- you and your doctor's responsibilities during the trial

You will also be assessed regularly for the four A's of pain medicine:

- **A**nalgesia (the inability to feel pain)
- **A**ctivity
- **A**dverse effects
- **A**berrant behaviors

There is now a fifth measure for **A**ffect, or how it moves a person emotionally. Frequency of assessment is determined by your level of risk.

A Closer Look

Some doctors may begin treatment by working their way up the World Health Organization's dated (1982–1986) pain analgesic ladder before prescribing opioids. However, keep in mind that this ladder was originally intended to make decisions about opioid trails with persons suffering from cancer pain.

World Health Organization Analgesic Ladder

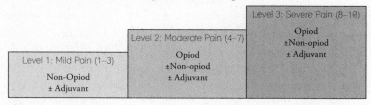

Level 1: Mild Pain (1–3)
Non-Opiod
± Adjuvant

Level 2: Moderate Pain (4–7)
Opiod
±Non-opiod
± Adjuvant

Level 3: Severe Pain (8–10)
Opiod
±Non-opiod
± Adjuvant

Tramadol

Tramadol is not considered an opioid. However, it is a short-acting medication to relieve pain that has weak activity at the opioid receptor. Tramadol also works as a serotonin-norepinephrine reuptake inhibitor (SNRI), similar to antidepressants. Tramadol was recently reclassified as schedule IV. Tramadol should not be used in people with a history of a seizure disorder. The dose must be adjusted for liver and kidney impairment. Caution should be used in people already on other serotonin medications which can increase the risk for serotonin syndrome when adding tramadol.

Adjuvants

Adjuvants are medication that enhance the effectiveness of medical treatment. These medications are indicated for the treatment of other conditions and have also been studied for the treatment of chronic neuropathic pain. The tricyclic antidepressants (TCAs) include amitriptyline, melipramine, and nortriptyline. TCAs are recommended for the treatment of diabetic neuropathy, post-herpetic neuralgia, migraine prophylaxis, and chronic low back pain. An adequate trial of an antidepressant for chronic pain is between four to eight weeks at a therapeutic dose. Unfortunately, many people are unable to tolerate TCAs due to side effects like

- sedation
- constipation
- urinary retention
- blurry vision
- dry mouth

TCAs should be used with caution in the elderly due to their increased risk for falls. TCAs should also be used with caution in people with cardiac histories due to the risk of chaotic heartbeats. It is recommended to obtain a baseline EKG for persons 40+ years old and limit the TCA dose to <100mg/day, if possible.

Serotonin-norepinephrine reuptake inhibitors (SNRIs) are also antidepressants recommended for the treatment of diabetic neuropathy. SNRIs have not been studied in post-herpetic neuralgia. SNRIs do not have the same side effects as the TCAs. Venlafaxine can be used for polyneuropathies and for migraine prophylaxis. Venlafaxine should be used with caution in people with heart disease due to the risk of conduction abnormalities. It can also cause dose-dependent increases in blood pressure, which should be monitored during therapy. Duloxetine is also indicated for the treatment of fibromyalgia and chronic musculoskeletal pain. The most common side effect associated with duloxetine is nausea, which can be minimized with slow addition till the target dose. Duloxetine is contraindicated in people with creatinine clearance <30ml/min or severe liver impairment. Milnacipran is another SNRI that is approved for the treatment of fibromyalgia. Since chronic pain and mood are directly related, many people are already on mood stabilizers. Thus, it is important to evaluate for potential drug interactions prior to starting an antidepressant for chronic pain.

Anticonvulsants are also recommended as first-line treatments for neuropathic conditions. Gabapentin and pregabalin are generally well tolerated. The common side effects include sedation, dizziness, dry mouth, weight gain, and edema. Pregabalin carries a warning to use with caution in people with Class III and IV heart failure. Both medications are started low and titrated as tolerated to target doses in order to minimize these side effects. Both also have to be dose adjusted for renal impairment. Pregabalin is also classified as a schedule V medication, indicating a risk of misuse and dependence. Gabapentin is cheaper, so it tends to be used more often. However, patients taking gabapentin will complain about how many pills they need to take at a time. For example, you may be started at 100mg TID (3 pills) and later escalated to 300mg TID (9 pills). Gabapentin is typically taken 3x/day because it only remains in your system for about 8 hours. This medication is not pain dependent, but rather must be maintained in order for it to be present in your system throughout a 24-hour period. More recently, there have been reports of patients abusing gabapentin.

Other anticonvulsants used for chronic pain include valproic acid and carbamazepine. Both require routine lab monitoring of liver function tests and complete blood counts for the duration of therapy. This is due to risk of thrombocytopenia and various anemias. People on carbamazepine are also routinely monitored for electrolyte imbalances, renal issues, skin reactions, thyroid, and eye effects. Carbamazepine is a potent CYP450 3A4 enzyme inducer, which can cause many multi-drug interactions. Persons initiated on an anticonvulsant for pain should be monitored closely for suicidal thoughts or symptoms of depression.

Steroids

Steroids are used to suppress inflammation and can help reduce pain. Examples of steroids include prednisone, methylprednisolone, and triamcinolone. Steroids can be prescribed for use orally, topically, or via injection. Steroids may be prescribed to treat a variety of conditions, including arthritis and muscle and disc inflammation. Side effects may include

- hyperglycemia
- increased risk of infections
- swelling
- risk for Cushing's Syndrome

Your doctor will determine if the long-term use of steroids is indicated based on whether the benefits outweigh the risks. You may be advised to alter your diet to reduce the amount of weight gained while on steroid medications. If you and your doctor determine to reduce or discontinue using steroids, you will be advised to do so gradually.

Topical Analgesics

Topical analgesics are available as creams, gels, sprays, liquid, patches, and balms OTC for the treatment of mild to moderate pain. Salicylate is an active ingredient in some topical analgesics that reduces pain and inflammation. Counterirritants are used for mild to moderate musculoskeletal pains associated with

- strains
- sprains
- back pain
- arthritis
- bruises

Topical analgesics can be applied several times a day to the affected area. Take care to avoid any wounds, damaged skin, or sensitive areas. People should be counseled to wash hands after application. Diclofenac is available as a prescription topical gel for the treatment of knee osteoarthritis. Capsaicin cream is used for both neuropathic pain and arthritis. The active ingredient is derived from hot peppers and can cause skin irritation and burning. People should be counseled to apply with gloves and wash hands after application. Capsaicin is also available as an 8% patch for the treatment of post-herpetic neuralgia. The patch must be administered in a doctor's office so you can be observed for response and tolerance. Lidocaine 5% patch is also FDA-approved for the treatment of post-herpetic neuralgia and localized central pain sensitization. Up to 3 patches may be applied in one setting for up to 12 hours, and the patches may be cut to fit.

Muscle Relaxants

Muscle relaxants are divided into two categories, antispastic and antispasmodic. Antipasti agents are used for the treatment of multiple sclerosis or cerebral palsy. There is limited evidence for their use in the treatment of musculoskeletal conditions. Muscle relaxants with antispasmodic properties can be used for the short-term treatment of acute pain. All muscle relaxants can cause dizziness and sedation. Cyclobenzaprine is structurally similar to TCAs and may have a similar mechanism of action and side effects. Cyclobenzaprine has been studied for use in low back pain and fibromyalgia. Carisoprodol is a schedule IV controlled substance because it is converted to meprobamate. This is a barbiturate-like drug that can cause both psychological and physical dependence. Selection of a muscle relaxant should be based on

- side effect profile
- abuse potential
- potential interactions
- patient specific information

There is limited evidence for long-term use of muscle relaxants for chronic pain and a lack of comparison data between muscle relaxants.

Medication management is just one component in an interdisciplinary treatment approach to chronic pain. Your doctor should discuss the risks and benefits and establish realistic treatment expectations with you prior to initiating a medication trial. Subsequent monitoring includes

- changes in pain severity
- effect on functionality
- progression towards defined goals
- occurrence of adverse side effects
- adherence to the recommended treatment plan
- the development of aberrant behaviors when applicable

Continuation of therapy should be re-evaluated periodically, and therapy tapered and discontinued if goals are not met, intolerable side effects occur, or aberrant behaviors persist.

A Quick Medication Guide

Non-Opiods	
Generic (Brand) Name	**Use**
Acetaminophen (Tylenol®)	Backache, headache, joint pain (arthritis), and muscle ache
Aspirin (Bayer®, Bufferin®)	Headache, joint pain and inflammation, muscle ache, and menstrual cramps
NSAIDs include the following: · Diclofenac (Voltaren®) · Ibuprofen (Advil®, Motrin®) · Meloxicam (Mobic®) · Naproxen (Aleve®, Naprosyn®) · COX-2 Inhibitors · Celecoxib (Celebrex®)	Arthritis pain and inflammation, backache, headache, menstrual cramps, muscle ache, and strains

Opiods	
Short-Acting Opioids: · Codeine/acetaminophen (Tylenol #3®) · Hydrocodone/acetaminophen · (Lortab®, Norco®, Vicodin®) · Oxycodone/acetaminophen (Percocet®) · Hydromorphone (Dilaudid®) · Morphine · Oxycodone (Roxicodone®) Long-Acting Opioids: · Fentanyl patches (Duragesic®) · Hydromorphone (Exalgo®) · Methadone (Dolophine®) · Morphine (Avinza®, Kadian®, MS Contin®) · Oxycodone (Oxycontin®) · Oxymorphone (Opana®)	Moderate to severe acute or chronic low back pain, osteoarthritis, and neuropathic pain after exhaustion of non-opioid and non-pharmacological therapies Evidence for efficacy in some types of chronic low back pain, daily headache, and fibromyalgia is limited
Tramadol (Ultram®)	Fibromyalgia, moderate to severe acute or chronic low back pain, neuropathic pain, and osteoarthritis

Adjuvants	
Tricyclic Antidepressants: · Amitriptyline (Elavil®) · Desipramine (Norpramin®) · Nortriptyline (Pamelor®)	Diabetic neuropathy, fibromyalgia, low back pain with radiculopathy, migraines, neuropathic pain, postherpetic neuralgia, and sympathetic dystrophy

Serotonin-Norepinephrine Reuptake Inhibitors: · Duloxetine (Cymbalta®) · Milnacipran (Savella®) · Venlafaxine (Effexor®)	Chronic musculoskeletal pain (duloxetine only), diabetic neuropathy (duloxetine and venlafaxine), fibromyalgia (duloxetine and milnacipran), migraines (venlafaxine), and neuropathic pain
Anticonvulsants: · Gabapentin (Neurontin®) · Pregabalin (Lyrica®)	Diabetic neuropathy, fibromyalgia, neuropathic pain, and post-herpetic neuralgia
Valproic acid (Depakote®)	Headache and neuropathic pain

Topical Analgesics

Capsaicin cream (Capzasin®, Zostrix®)	Neuropathic pain, osteoarthritis, rheumatoid arthritis
Capsaicin 8% patch (Qutenza®)	Post-herpetic neuralgia
Diclofenac Topical Gel (Voltaren®)	Osteoarthritis
Lidocaine 5% patches (Lidoderm®)	Allodynia and post-herpetic neuralgia
Menthol/Salicylate (BenGay®, Icy Hot®, Salonpas®, Thera-Gesic®)	Arthritis, back pain, sprains and strains

Muscle Relaxants

Carisoprodol (Soma®) Cyclobenzaprine (Flexeril®) Metaxalone (Skelaxin®) Methocarbamol (Robaxin®) Tizanidine (Zanaflex®)	Acute (less than two weeks) low back pain and fibromyalgia (cyclobenzaprine)

A Patient Story

A 68-year-old male goes to a pain clinic for the first time reporting neck and lower back pain. He has suffered from pain since the 1960s after several car accidents. He discusses at length all the various opioids he has been on throughout the years with his doctor. He also shares that he has repeatedly been able to "wean himself off" opioids in past. He is in the pain clinic hoping that a 30-day supply of fentanyl patches could be prescribed. He expects that the opioid should help considering his history.

 Is it the medications alone that accounts for the outcome or are there other factors to consider in this outcome? The answers are discussed in chapter 7.

Summary of the Research

Medication management will continue to be the backbone of chronic pain treatment. The classes of drugs most commonly used for the treatment of chronic, non-cancer pain are

- opioids
- NSAIDs
- antidepressants
- anticonvulsants
- muscle relaxants
- topical agents

A combination of results from several studies have concluded that

- opioids result in small improvements in pain severity and function compared with placebo
- antidepressants result in moderate symptom reduction and are superior to placebo

The efficacy of NSAIDs has been established for some patients with pain, but has not been investigated in others. The best evidence supports the efficacy of anticonvulsant drugs for the treatment of chronic, non-cancer pain. Muscle relaxants are typically recommended as adjuvant therapy and seem to have a restricted role in chronic pain. Topical agents have also been shown to effectively reduce chronic pain in comparison to placebo.

Interventions

Intervention approaches are advanced medical procedures that are performed, often through penetration of the skin. Interventions include

- epidural steroid injections
- nerve blocks
- trigger point injections
- neurostimulation
- surgery

The decision of which intervention is used is based on pain severity or persistence or how bothersome the pain is. Your doctor will determine which modality to recommend based on these indices and how invasive the therapy will be.

Epidural Steroid Injections

Epidural steroid injections (ESIs) are the most widely utilized pain management procedure in the world. ESIs deliver anti-inflammatory medication into the epidural space of the spine using X-ray guidance. ESIs are used to alleviate chronic pain in the lower back (lumbar or LESI), mid-back (thoracic or TESI), and neck (cervical or CESI). More localized procedures, such as caudal and transforaminal ESIs, help reduce lower chronic back pain that radiates down the leg. ESIs are often performed in a procedural clinic, usually with the patient lying face down on a fluoroscopy table. Numbing medicine and then contrast dye is injected into the site. Using x-ray guidance, the doctor then places the steroid medication into the specific epidural space. The procedure takes about 15 minutes. The exact timing varies by clinical practice. The patient is then observed for 20 to 30 minutes before being driven home by a companion. Although rare, patients may suffer from headaches after an ESI, which may require a blood patch. Neurological complications (such as stroke and paralysis) have been associated with ESIs but are extremely rare.

A Closer Look

The human spine can be broken down into several different sections: skull (cranium), neck (cervical), mid-back (thoracic), lower back (lumbar), and sacrum (tailbone). Interventions can be performed at all levels of the spine.

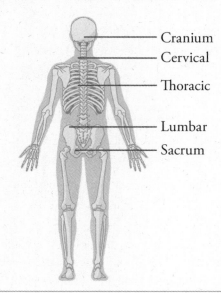

Cranium
Cervical
Thoracic
Lumbar
Sacrum

Facet Injections

Facet joint injections involve injecting a small amount of local anesthetic or steroid medication at the cervical, thoracic, or lumbar facet joint. They can anesthetize the facet joints and block the pain. Multiple injections may be performed depending upon how many joints are involved. A facet joint injection is usually performed in a procedural clinic. They are best performed using fluoroscopy for guidance to properly target and place the needle. This practice helps avoid nerve injury or other injury. The patient typically rests for 20 to 30 minutes, and then is asked to perform some movements that would provoke their pain. You may or may not obtain pain relief in the first few hours after the injection. It depends upon whether the joints targeted are the main source of your pain. If the joint or joints being targeted are not causing the pain, you will not obtain immediate relief from injection.

Nerve Blocks

A nerve block is an injection directly around the nerves that serve an area of pain, including occipital and sympathetic. A medial branch block (MBB) is a diagnostic injection that temporarily interrupts the pain signal being carried from a specific facet joint. If the MBB proves to be successful, then a radio-frequency nerve ablation may be performed. Radio frequency waves are used to produce heat on specifically identified nerves surrounding the facet joints. You may take your medications with a small amount of water, except if taking any blood thinners. These medications must be discontinued well before the procedure with your doctor's consent. Nerve blocks are often performed in a procedural clinic, usually with the patient lying on their stomach on a fluoroscopy table. The site of the nerve block is then cleaned with an anti-bacterial solution. Numbing medicine is injected into the site, and x-ray imaging is used to guide placement of the needle. The patient is then observed for 30 to 45 minutes before being driven home by a companion. Complications due to the nerve block are rare but can include infection, bleeding, or an injection into a blood vessel.

A Quick Injection/Procedure Guide

Type	Indications
Lumbar epidural steroid injection (ESI) Interlaminar	· Radicular pain from herniated discs, degenerative disc disease (irritation nerve root) · spinal canal stenosis
Caudal ESI	· Radicular pain as mentioned above, prior posterior lumbar instrumentation or surgery (laminectomy with scarring) · Severe degenerative disc disease, narrow vertebral interspace, mineralized ligaments

Lumbar ESI Transforaminal	· Radicular pain—one-sided · More reliable for delivery to specific nerve roots · Loss of resistance may not be reliable with history of prior back surgery, scarring, reduced epidural space
Sacroiliac Joint Injection	· Sacroiliac joint dysfunction · Dull aching pain over buttock/anterolateral thigh & groin · May be used as a diagnostic measure · Sacroiliac joint tenderness and positive exam
Lumbar Medial Branch Block (MBB)	· Centralized (somatic) low back pain · Limited extension to low extremities · Localized tenderness at facet joints or paraspinal muscles · Facet Arthropathy
Lumbar Radiofrequency Nerve Ablation (RFA)	· Centralized (somatic) low back pain · Facet Arthropathy · Appropriate response to MBB

Trigger Point Injections

Trigger point injections are a series of local anesthetic shots administered in specific areas of the muscle. These areas of the muscle are pain generators. The trigger point injection is often performed in the doctor's office. Usually the patient either lies on the exam table on their stomach or sits on the exam table. The exact protocol varies by clinical practice setting. The doctor performing the procedure locates the trigger point by manual palpation and marks the site. The injection site is then cleaned with alcohol or another skin cleanser. After the injection, a simple adhesive bandage may be applied.

Spinal Cord Stimulators

Spinal cord stimulation (SCS) is used to treat chronic and intractable pain, including

- failed back surgery syndrome
- complex regional pain syndrome
- phantom limb pain

A simple SCS system consists of three different parts:

1. microelectrodes (implanted in the epidural space to deliver stimulation pulses to the spinal cord)

2. an electrical pulse generator (implanted in the lower abdominal area or gluteal region while is connected to the electrodes via wires)
3. a remote control (to adjust the stimulus parameters such as pulse width and pulse rate)

Candidates for the SCS must undergo a medical and psychological evaluation, a trial procedure for a week, a final implant surgery, and follow-up with a gradual decrease of medications.

Intrathecal Drug Delivery Systems

An intrathecal drug delivery system (IDDS) delivers pain medication directly to the fluid around the spinal cord, or the intrathecal space. The system includes a drug pump that is connected to a thin, flexible tube called a catheter. Both the pump and the catheter are fully implanted under the skin. Because the pump releases medication to receptors near the spine, pain relief can be achieved with a small fraction of the oral medication dose. Currently there are only three medications approved by the US Food and Drug Administration (FDA) for use via the intrathecal route, including morphine, ziconotide, and baclofen.

Surgery

In terms of surgery, evidence has rated lumber fusion as "fair," and both discectomy and laminectomy as "good." This is with the provision that significant pain can persist even after spinal surgery. Patients at times will express concern that they continue to have pain after surgery. My response is usually "yes, that is to be expected. Imagine that your doctor told you the surgery would only be 60% successful. That would mean that you would still have 40% of your pain remaining." If this same patient comes to the pain clinic and reports their pain as a "5," that is around the amount that is expected to remain. The patient will need to continue to be engaged in pain management.

A Patient Story

A 69-year-old male returns to the pain clinic after having a medial blanch block for arthritis in his joints of his spine about six months ago. The patient reports that he continues to have relief from the MBB, which is similar to the outcomes he has had in the past with other injections. The relief from the MBB should have only lasted a couple of hours.

 Was it the injection/procedure alone that accounts for the outcome or are there other factors to consider in this outcome? The answers are discussed in chapter 7.

Summary of the Research

Interventional pain medicine involves the application of various techniques, such as

- injections
- implantable devices
- surgery

Epidural steroid and facet injections are the most commonly used in the United States. However, the evidence for epidural steroid injection use as long-term monotherapy is not clear. Facet injections have some evidence for use with facet joint pain, but are not clearly successful for other syndromes. A combination of results from several studies have evaluated the efficacy of SCS. They concluded that there was moderate evidence for improvement in pain with SCS. A more recent systematic review evaluated the success of IDDS and determined that there were moderate reductions in pain but unclear long-term success.

Physical Medicine & Rehabilitation

Physical medicine and rehabilitation (PM&R), or physiatry, is a branch of medicine. PM&R aims to enhance and restore functional ability and quality of life to those with physical impairments/disabilities. Chronic pain management is achieved through a multidisciplinary approach involving

- physical therapists
- occupational therapists
- exercise therapists

Exercise will be covered in more detail later in chapter 5. Back pain has been estimated to account for 45% of all physiatry visits and is one of the most expensive injuries to treat. Rehabilitation, specifically for low back pain, occurs in three phases:

1. Physiatrists make a specific diagnosis, develop a treatment plan, and offer treatment options
2. Flexibility and strength are developed to get the body parts into their proper positions
3. A total-body fitness program is designed to maintain body mechanics and increase endurance

Using Good Body Mechanics

Body mechanics is a term used to describe the way you move throughout the day. Poor body mechanics are often the cause of back problems. When you move incorrectly and not safely, the spine is subjected to abnormal stresses. Over time, this can lead to degeneration of spinal structures like discs and joints, injury, and unnecessary wear and tear. That is why it is so important to learn about proper body mechanics. Proper body mechanics maintain the natural curve of the spine. The spine normally curves at the neck, the torso, and the lower back area. This positions the head over the pelvis naturally. The curves also work as shock absorbers, distributing the stress that occurs during movement. When the spine curves too far inward, the condition is called swayback. Good posture means the spine is in a neutral position. It includes how you hold the body when lifting, standing/walking, driving, sitting, and sleeping.

A Closer Look

But what does good posture look like?

You can use the following five steps:

1. Stand with the feet apart
2. Tuck the tailbone in and tilt the pelvic bone slightly forward
3. Pull the shoulders back and lift the chest
4. Lift the chin until it is level
5. Relax the jaw and mouth

Lifting: The process of lifting places perhaps the greatest loads on the low back and has the highest risk of injury. Use of proper lifting mechanics and posture is critical to prevent injury. You must bend with the knees, not the back, when lifting. Do not bend over with the legs straight or twist while lifting. You must lift with the legs and hold objects close to the body. Lift objects only chest-high and stand on a stool if necessary. Avoid trying to lift above the shoulder level. When a load is heavy, get help and plan ahead to avoid sudden load shifts. It is always important that you are sure about your footing. In the end, it is more important how you lift than how heavy a weight you lift.

Standing/Walking: Millions of people spend a good deal of their time on their feet. Standing can be tough on the back, especially if proper body mechanics are not being used. You should stand with weight on one foot and change positions often. Do not stand in one position too long. Stand with the back's three natural curves in their normal, balanced alignment as explained previously. Walk with good posture, keeping the head held high, chin tucked in, and toes pointed straight ahead. Do not bend forward with straight legs or walk with poor posture. Wear comfortable, low-heeled shoes. Do not wear high-heeled or platform shoes when standing or walking for long periods.

Driving: According to a study done by the Harvard Health Watch, an average American spends 101 minutes per day driving. You should move the car seat forward to keep knees level with the hips. Do not drive far back from the steering wheel. Stretching for the pedals and wheel decreases the lower back's curve and produces strain. Sit straight and drive with both hands on the steering wheel. To support the lower back, you may place a lumbar support or a rolled-up towel behind the back.

Sitting: Whether sitting at a computer desk or at home watching television, good body mechanics are still important to keep in mind. A study done in 2010 found that an average American spends 32 hours per month online. According to the U.S. Bureau of Labor Statistics, the average American watches TV for 2.8 hours per day. You must sit in chairs that are low enough to place both feet flat on the floor with the knees level with the hips. Do not sit in a chair that is too high or too far from the desk. Avoid leaning forward and arching the back. Adjust the computer screen to eye level to avoid additional neck strain. Sit firmly against the back of the chair. Do not slump. Protect the lower back with a lumbar support or rolled-up towel. Keep in mind that even sitting with good posture for long periods of time will eventually become uncomfortable. Do not forget to take breaks, get up, move around, and stretch approximately every 30–45 minutes. These behaviors will reduce the stress on your spine and help prevent muscle fatigue and stiffness.

Sleeping: People on average sleep for 8 hours a day. A good night's sleep on a firm mattress is good for the back. Use a pillow that keeps the head aligned with the rest of the body. Numerous and/or oversized pillows may look great on a made bed but do not necessarily benefit the back while sleeping. Do not sleep or lounge on soft, sagging, non-supporting mattresses or cushions. People should be informed about mattress flipping and the need to update their mattress after four years, which is considered optimal. It is recommended to sleep on your side with the knees bent and a pillow between them, or on the back with a pillow under the knees. Swayback and back strain will result when sleeping on the stomach. Choose the position that feels the most comfortable.

A Quick Body Posture Guide

DO	DON'T
Lifting	
· Bend with your knees · Lift with your legs and hold objects close to your body · Lift objects chest-high · Stand on a stool if necessary · Ask for help if load is heavy · Plan ahead to avoid sudden load shifts · Be sure of footing	· Bend with your back · Bend over with legs straight · Twist while lifting · Lift above shoulder level
Standing/Walking	
· Stand with weight on one foot · Change positions often · Stand with three natural curves in alignment · Walk with good posture · Wear comfortable low-heeled shoes	· Stand in one position too long · Bend forward with straight legs · Walk with poor posture · Wear high-heeled or platform shoes when standing or walking for long periods
Driving	
· Move car seat forward to keep knees level with hips · Sit straight · Drive with both hands on the wheel · Place a lumbar support or rolled-up towel behind your back	· Drive sitting far back from the wheel · Stretch for pedals and wheel (decreases low back curve and produces strain)
Sitting	
· Sit in chairs low enough to place both feet flat on the floor with knees level with hips · Sit firmly against the back of your chair · Protect your lower back with lumbar support or rolled-up towel	· Slump · Sit in a chair that's too high or too far from your desk · Leaning forward and arching your back
Sleeping	
· Sleep on a firm mattress · Sleep on your side with your knees bent or on your back with a pillow under your knees · Choose the position that feels more comfortable to you	· Sleep or lounge on soft, sagging, non-supporting mattresses or cushions · Sleep on your stomach-that can result in swayback and back strain

Self-Care Aids

Due to a disability or after sustaining an injury, you may find it difficult to perform activities of daily living (ADLs). ADLs include bathing, dressing, grooming/hygiene, toileting, and feeding. Occupational therapists can help you develop skills needed to complete your ADLs as independently as possible. It may also be necessary to use adaptive equipment, devices that are used to assist with completing ADLs. Past studies have shown that this equipment is about 88% used and 85% considered beneficial for chronic lower back pain in hospitals. This was associated with the number of occupational therapy sessions provided. Studies have shown there are five factors that predict whether patients are compliant with this equipment when prescribed for home use, including

1. medical related (diagnosis or other medical condition)
2. client related (age, gender, and satisfaction of equipment)
3. equipment related (suitability, replacement, and delivery)
4. assessment related (adequate assessment and home visits)
5. training related (frequency of sessions and training of caregiver)

The following examples of adaptive equipment are commonly prescribed to patients who suffer from chronic pain. This is just a small sampling of the equipment that may be used to increase independence.

Bathing: In the first few days or weeks following injury, you may not be able to bathe regularly and may take sponge baths in bed. The occupational therapist can help you learn how to shower safely using a long-handled sponge or a shower chair. This is once you are medically stable and cleared for showering by your doctor. The long-handled sponge is designed for use by individuals with upper extremity or mobility disabilities or limited range of motion. The sponge can come in different shapes and is covered in plastic. Make sure to take the plastic off before using the sponge! A shower chair is usually a sturdy seat made from corrosion resistant aluminum tubing. It has a curved, textured plastic seat with handles and drain holes to allow easy and safe transfer. The legs are fitted with anti-slip, non-marking rubber feet.

Dressing: Upper body dressing includes putting on and taking off any clothing items from the waist up. For most individuals, the upper extremities are usually functioning properly and upper body dressing is completed without difficulty. Lower body dressing includes putting on and taking off any clothing item from the waist down. When dressing the lower body, persons with pain might find it helpful to use a combination of adaptive equipment. The most common position for performing lower body dressing is sitting in bed. This allows the person to maintain balance. Some of the most common pieces of adaptive equipment used during dressing include a pick-up stick, the long-handled shoe horn, the sock remover, elastic shoelaces, the sock lead, and the leg grip. The "reacher," or pick-up stick, can help you pick up objects up to 5 pounds off the floor without straining their back. It can also be used to reach items on the top shelf of the cupboard. The long-handled shoe horn reduces the need to bend when putting on shoes or slippers. It features a handle grip providing a comfortable hold. The function of the sock remover is its namesake. You can also use elastic shoelaces to turn any shoes into slip-ons. You will never have to tie laces again when using curly elastic shoelaces. Simply thread the curly laces in, pull them snug, and shoes are always ready to put on. The sock lead, or "stocking aid," allows you to put your socks or stockings on with ease. Ideally, the sock lead is for those who have difficulty bending at the waist. You hold your sock or stocking firmly in place while pulling them around your foot. Finally, the leg grip, or "lift strap," is a simple but practical leg lifter that is useful for people with limited lower extremity strength. It enables you to lift the foot onto a wheelchair foot rest, bed, or into a car. It is also used to stretch the hamstrings while in physical therapy.

Grooming/Hygiene: Grooming tasks include brushing teeth, washing face, combing hair, shaving, and applying makeup. As with upper body dressing, most individuals usually have full use of their arms and grooming is completed without difficulty. This is done from a chair as long as items are in reach. For other people, grooming becomes more difficult and is completed in a supported, seated position in bed or a wheelchair. Once you can tolerate a sitting position, the occupational therapist will help you practice techniques to complete these activities. This will be done as independently as possible using adaptive equipment, such as a foot brush and an inspection mirror. The foot brush and the inspection mirror are designed for use by individuals with diabetes, mobility disabilities, or arthritis. The foot brush comes with a sponge that you can use for cleaning between toes and applying medication.

Toileting: Toileting includes the ability to pull down clothing, clean the rectal/genital areas, and pull clothing up. A person is often able to independently complete the process with the correct technique and needed equipment. Toileting for some individuals is usually difficult. The occupational therapist will develop a specialized toileting program for patients/caregivers for home use. Adaptive equipment may include a toilet tissue aid. This aid is a simple solution for people who need an extended reach to their rectal/genital area. The spring clamp on this toilet tissue holder easily opens to release tissue paper. This bathroom aid is ideal for persons who are disabled, obese, or small in stature.

Feeding: Feeding, like upper body dressing and grooming, is usually not difficult for most individuals. Feeding is usually done in a supported seated position in bed with a bedside table or from wheelchair level with a lap tray. There are several pieces of adaptive equipment available to assist with this process, including adaptive utensils, scoop dishes, long-handled straws, one-handed cutting boards, and can openers.

The adaptive devices reviewed above differ from medical equipment. Medical equipment is designed to aid in the diagnosis, monitoring, or treatment of medical conditions. There are several basic types of medical equipment, including

1. diagnostic (ultrasound and x-ray)
2. treatment (infusion pumps)
3. life support (ventilators and dialysis machines)
4. medical monitors (blood pressure)
5. medical laboratory (blood and urine analyses)
6. therapeutic (transcutaneous electrical nerve stimulation units)

Only two types of equipment will be covered in more detail: transcutaneous electric nerve stimulation units and other electrical stimulation devices.

A Quick Self-Care Aid Guide

Adaptive Equipment	Purpose	Example
Sponge with Long Handle	· Used for bathing · Make sure you take the plastic off before using it	
Shower Seat	· Used for bathing · Made from corrosion resistant aluminum tubing · Plastic seat with handles and drain holes to allow easy and safe transfer · Legs are fitted with antislip non-marking rubber feet	
Pick-up Stick or "The Reacher"	· Helps pick up objects off the floor · Can pick up to 5 pounds · Can also be used to reach items on top shelf	
Leg Grip/Lift Strap	· Leg lifter useful with limited lower extremity strength · Lift the foot onto a wheelchair foot rest, onto a bed, or into a car · Used to stretch hamstrings in PT	

Long-handled Shoe Horn and Elastic Shoelaces	· Reduces the need to bend · Features a handle grip · Never tie laces again · Laces turn any shoes into slip-ons	
Sock Remover and Sock Lead or Stocking Aid	· Ideal for those who have difficulty bending at the waist · Holds socks and stockings firmly in place while pulling them around the foot	
Foot Brush & Inspection Mirror	· For use by diabetics and arthritics · Sponges used for cleaning toes and applying medication · Mirror useful to inspect for cuts or infections on the bottom of feet	
Toilet Paper Holder	· Simple solution for an extended reach · Clamp on holder easily opens to release tissue paper · Ideal for obese or small people	
Adaptive Utensils and Dishes	· Feeding is usually done in a supported seated position in bed with a bedside table or from wheelchair level with a lap tray · There are several pieces of adaptive equipment, including adaptive utensils, scoop dishes, long-handled straws, one-handed cutting boards, and can openers	

Transcutaneous Electric Nerve Stimulation (TENS) Unit

A typical battery-operated TENS unit is a device that applies currents to the outer layer of the skin through two or more electrodes. TENS are used for nerve excitation to suppress pain. In principle, an adequate intensity of stimulation is necessary to achieve pain relief with TENS. People report the sensation as strong but comfortable. Evidence supporting the use of TENS has been inconsistent. One review provided evidence that TENS use with chronic musculoskeletal pain was beneficial. Another study deemed the evidence was of poor quality and thus no conclusions were possible. Other studies have found no clinically significant benefit to TENS for the treatment of neck pain or chronic low back pain. There is tentative evidence that it may be helpful for diabetic neuropathy. More recently, a head-mounted TENS device, Cefaly®, was approved by the US FDA in 2014 for the prevention of migraines.

Electrical Stimulation

TENS devices differ from cranial electrotherapy stimulation (CES) or microcurrent electrical therapy (MET). TENS applies electrical currents on the surface of peripheral nerve route sites on the extremities or other non-cranial areas. It is the distinct waveform of the CES and MET that differentiates them from other devices. Electrical stimulation treatments are relatively safe and easy to use, and they have research evidence to support their success in treating fibromyalgia. CES devices deliver modified square-wave biphasic stimulation at 0.5Hz and 100uA through the electrodes placed on the ear lobes. An average CES session lasts between 20 and 60 minutes. Research has also indicated that the use of MET can complement or improve results of the CES. MET is provided directly to the body either through handheld probe electrodes or self-adhesive electrodes. The probes of the MET device are repositioned every 10 seconds following a beep from the device. They are placed through the area of the pain complaint. The Alpha-Stim® devices are FDA approved for the treatment of pain (MET) and depression, anxiety, and insomnia (CES). Side effects from CES and MET include vertigo, headache, nausea, and skin irritation at the site of the electrodes in <1% of patients. Caution is advised during pregnancy and with patients with older pacemaker models circa 1998. It is also not recommended that patients operate complex machinery or automobiles during the treatment.

A Patient Story

A 68-year-old male suffering from early stages of Parkinson's disease goes to the pain clinic in a motorized wheelchair accompanied by his son. Since he has been coming to the pain clinic, he has had physical and occupational therapy at home. The patient and his son feel this has made a significant improvement in pain, strength, and coordination. The patient has exhausted the 12 sessions covered by his insurance. He is now requesting further visits at home if it can get approved due to barriers in his son's social situation.

 Was it the physical and occupational therapy alone that account for the outcome or are there other factors to consider in this outcome? The answers are discussed in chapter 7.

Summary of the Research

Evidence suggests that exercise can effectively decrease pain and improve function, but no conclusions can be made about exercise type. Physical medicine approaches are commonly included as components of interdisciplinary pain rehabilitation programs. The use of proper body mechanics and self-care aids is recommended for people who suffer from chronic pain, especially during rehabilitation.

Conclusion

In chapter 3, I reviewed the traditional approaches to chronic pain management, including medications, interventions, and physical medicine and rehabilitation modalities. I continue to explore options for treatment in the next chapter on psychological interventions, specifically meditation, acceptance and commitment therapy, biofeedback, relaxation techniques, cognitive-behavioral therapy, and hypnosis.

References

Aeschbach A, Mekhail N. (2000). Common nerve blocks in chronic pain management. *Anesthesiology Clinics of North America*, 18, 429–459.

American Chronic Pain Association. Resource Guide to Chronic Pain and Treatment 2015 Edition. Available at: http://www.theacpa.org/uploads/documents/ACPA_Resource_Guide_2015_Final%20edited%20(3).pdf. Accessed: 4/30/15.

Armon, C., Argoff, C., Samuels, J., & Backonja, M. (2007). Assessment: Use of epidural steroid injections to treat radicular lumbosacral pain: A report of the Therapeutics and Technology Assessment Subcommittee of the American Academy of Neurology. Neurology, 68, 723–729.

Arnold, L., Keck, P., & Welge, J. (2000). Antidepressant treatment of fibromyalgia: A meta-analysis and review. *Psychosomatics*, 41, 104–13.

Attal, N., Cruccu, G., Baron, R., et al. (2010). EFNS guidelines on the pharmacological treatment of neuropathic pain: 2010 revision. *European Journal of Neurology*, 17, 1113–e88.

Ballantyne JC and Mao J. Opioid Therapy for Chronic Pain. *N Engl J Med* 2003; 349:1943–53.

Ballantyne JC and Shin NS. Efficacy of opioids for chronic pain: a review of the evidence. *Clin J Pain* 2008; 24:469–478.

Bateman B, Brenner G. (2015). An important step forward in the safe use of epidural steroid injections. *Anesthesiology*, 122, 964–966.

Battié M, Crites M, Cherkin D, et al. (1994). Managing low back pain: Attitudes and treatment Preferences of physical therapists. *Physical Therapy Journal*, 74, 219–226.

Better Sleep Council. A New Mattress Does the Body Good. Available at: http://bettersleep.org/better-sleep/healthy-sleep/physical-performance-sleep. Accessed 3/31/15.

Bril V, England J, Franklin GM, et al. Evidence-based guideline: treatment of painful diabetic neuropathy, report of the American Academy of Neurology, the American Association of Neuromuscular and Electrodiagnostic Medicine, and the American Academy of Physical Medicine and Rehabilitation. *Neurology* 2011; 76:1–8.

Chou R, Fanciullo GJ, Fine PG. Clinical guidelines for the use of chronic opioid therapy in chronic noncancer pain. *J Pain* 2009; 10(2):113–130.

Chou R, Qaseem A, Snow V, Casey D, Cross T, Shekelle P, Owens D. Diagnosis and treatment of low back pain: A Joint Clinical Practice Guideline from the America College of Physicians and the American Pain Society. *Ann Intern Med*. 2007; 147:478–491.

Chou, R., Atlas, S., Stanos, S., & Rosenquist, R. (2009). Nonsurgical interventional therapies for low back pain. *Spine*, 34, 1078–1093.

Chou, R., Baisden, J., Carragee, E., et al. (2009). Surgery for low back pain: A review of the evidence for an American Pain Society Clinical Practice Guideline. *Spine*, 34, 1094–1109.

Chou, R., Loeser, J., Owens, D., et al. (2009). Interventional therapies, surgery, and interdisciplinary rehabilitation for low back pain. *Spine*, 34, 1066–1077.

Cohe S, Bicket M, Jamison D, et al. (2013). Epidural steroids: A comprehensive, evidence-based review. *Regional Anesthesia and Pain Medicine*, 38, 175–200.

Colorado Comprehensive Spine Institute. The importance of proper body mechanics-Keeping your spine healthy. Available at: http://www.coloradospineinstitute.com/subject.php?pn=wellness-body-mechanics. Accessed May 11, 2015.

Cork, R., Wood, P., Ming, N., et al. (2003). The effect of cranial electrotherapy stimulation (CES) on pain associated with fibromyalgia. *The Internet Journal of Anesthesiology*, 8.

DeBerard, M., Masters, K., Colledge, A., Schleusener, R., & Schlegel, J. (2001). Outcomes of posterolateral lumbar fusion in Utah patients receiving workers' compensation: A retrospective cohort study. *Spine*, 26, 738–746.

Drug Enforcement Administration. Schedules of controlled substances: placement of tramadol into schedule IV. Department of Justice. 2014;79(127). Available at: http://www.deadiversion.usdoj.gov/fed_regs/rules/2014/fr0702.htm. Accessed 5/12/15.

Dubinsky R, Miyasaki J. (2009). Assessment: Efficacy of transcutaneous electric nerve stimulation in the treatment of pain in neurologic disorders (an evidence-based review). *Neurology*, 74, 173–176.

Dworkin RH, O'Connor AB, Audette J, et al. Recommendations for the pharmacological management of neuropathic pain: an overview and literature update. *Mayo Clin Proc*. 2010; 85(3)(suppl):S3–S14.

Family Friendly Fun. Adaptive Equipment. Available at: http://www.family-friendly-fun.com/disabilities/adaptive-equipment.htm. Accessed May 11. 2105.

Finnerup, N., Sindrup, S., & Jensen, T. (2010). The evidence for pharmacological treatment of neuropathic pain. *Pain*, 150, 573–581.

Franklin GM. Opioids for chronic noncancer pain: a position paper of the American Academy of Neurology. *Neurology*, 2014; 83:1277–1284.

Frey, M., Manchikanti, L., Benyamin, R., et al. (2009). Spinal cord stimulation for patients with failed back surgery syndrome: A systematic review. *Pain Physician*, 12, 379–397.

Friedly, J., Nishio, I., Bishop, M., & Maynard, C. (2008). The relationship between repeated epidural steroid injections and subsequent opioid use and lumbar surgery. *Archives of Physical Medicine & Rehabilitation*, 89, 1011–1015.

Furlan, A., Sandoval, J., Mailis-Gagnon, A., & Tunks, E. (2006). Opioids for chronic non-cancer pain: A meta-analysis of effectiveness and side effects. *Canadian Medical Association Journal*, 174, 1589–1594.

Galer B, Argoff C. (2010). *Defeat Chronic Pain Now!* Fair Wind Press: Beverly, MA.

Glajchen M. (2001). Chronic pain: Treatment barriers and strategies for clinical practice. *Journal of the American Board of Family Practice*, 14, 211–218.

Gourlay DL, Heit HL, Almahrezi A. Universal precautions in pain medicine: a rational approach to the treatment of chronic pain. *Pain Med*. 2005;6(2):107–12.

Haldeman S, Carroll L, Cassidy J, et al. (2008). The bone and joint decade 2000–2010 task force on neck pain and its associated disorders. *Spine*, 33, S5–S7.

Hornberger, J., Kumar, K., Verhulst, E., Clark, M., & Hernandez, J. (2008). Rechargeable spinal cord stimulation versus non-rechargeable system for patients with failed back surgery syndrome: A cost-consequences analysis. *Clinical Journal of Pain*, 24, 244–252.

Hospital for Special Surgery. What is Physiatry? Available at: http://www.hss.edu/what-is-physiatry.asp#. VVDo_DYcS2w. Accessed May 11, 2015.

International Association for the Study of Pain. IASP Taxonomy. Available at: http://www.iasp-pain. org/ Taxonomy. Accessed May 22, 2012.

Johnson M, Martinson M. (2007). Efficacy of electrical nerve stimulation for chronic musculoskeletal pain: A meta-analysis of randomized controlled trials. *Pain*, 130, 157–165.

Keller, A., Hayden, J., Bombardier, C., & van Tulder, M. (2007). Effect sizes of non-surgical treatments of non-specific low-back pain. *European Spine Journal*, 16, 1776–1788.

Khadilkar A, Odebiyi D, Brosseau L, et al. (2008). Transcutaneous electrical nerve stimulation (TENS) versus placebo for chronic low-back pain. The Cochrane Library. Available at: http://onlinelibrary.wiley. com/doi/10.1002/14651858.CD003008.pub3/abstract.

Kirsch, D. & Marksberry, J. (2015). The evolution of cranial electrotherapy stimulation for anxiety, insomnia, depression and pain and its potential for other indications. In: Rosch, P. (2015). *Bioelectromagnetic and Subtle Energy Medicine (2nd ed)*. Boca Raton, FL: CRC Press.

Kroenke, K., Krebs, E., & Bair, M. (2009). Pharmacotherapy of chronic pain: A synthesis of recommendations from systematic reviews. *General Hospital Psychiatry*, 31, 206–219.

Kulkarni, A. (2001). The use of microcurrent electrical therapy and cranial electrotherapy stimulation in pain control. *Clinical Practice of Alternative Medicine*, 2, 99–102.

Lanza Fl, Chan K, Eamon Q, and the Practice Parameters Committee of the American College of Gastroenterology. Guidelines for prevention of NSAID-related ulcer complications. *Am J Gastroenterol*. 2009; 104:728–738.

Lichtbroun, A., Raicer, M., & Smith, R. (2001). The treatment of fibromyalgia with cranial electrotherapy stimulation. *Journal of Clinical Rheumatology*, 7, 72–78.

Luijsterburg, P., Verhagen, A., Ostelo, R., et al. (2007). Effectiveness of conservative treatments for the lumbosacral radicular syndrome: A systematic review. *European Spine Journal*, 16, 881–899.

Manchikanti, L. (2004). The growth of interventional pain management in the new millennium: A critical analysis of utilization in the Medicare population. *Pain Physician*, 7, 465–482.

Mason, L., Moore, R., Edwards, J., et al. (2004). Systematic review of efficacy of topical rubefacients containing salicylates for the treatment of acute and chronic pain. *British Medical Journal*, 328, 995.

Mercola, J. & Kirsch, D. (1995). The basis for microcurrent electrical therapy in conventional medicine practice. *Journal of Advanced Medicine* , 8, 107–120.

Neal C. (1997). The assessment of knowledge and application of proper body mechanics in the workplace. *Orthopedic Nursing*, 16, PDF Only.

Nnoaham K, Kumbang J. (2008). Transcutaneous electrical nerve stimulation (TENS) for chronic pain. The Cochrane Library. Available at: http://onlinelibrary.wiley.com/doi/10.1002/14651858.CD003222. pub2/abstract;jsessionid=25D76FB0AD19E78B41100B1DF9EDCF4E.f03t03.

Robertson V, Ward A, Low J, et al. (2006). *Electrotherapy explained: Principles and practice (4th ed.)*. Butterworth-Heinemann (Elsevier).

Roelofs, P., Deyo, R., Koes, B., Scholten, R., & van Tulder, M. (2008). Non-steroidal anti-inflammatory drugs for low back pain. *Cochrane Database of Systematic Reviews*, 1.

Schoenen J, Vandersmissen B, Jeangette S, et al. (2013). Migraine prevention with a supraorbital transcutaneous stimulator: A randomized controlled trial. *Neurology*, 80, 697–704.

See S and Ginzburg R. Choosing a skeletal muscle relaxant. Am Fam Physician. 2008; 78(3):365–370.

Silberstein SD, Holland S, Freitag F, et al. Evidence-baseline guideline update: pharmacologic treatment of episodic migraine prevention in adults, report of the Quality Standards Subcommittee of the American Academy of Neurology and the American Headache Society. *Neurology* 2012; 78:1337–1345.

Singh, G. & Triadafilopoulos, G. (1999). Epidemiology of NSAID induced gastrointestinal complications. *Journal of Rheumatology Supplement*, 56, 18–24.

Taylor, A., Anderson, J, Riedel, S., et al. (2013). A randomized, controlled, double-blind pilot study of the effects of cranial electrical stimulation on activity in brain pain processing regions in individuals with fibromyalgia. *Explore*, 9, 32–40.

Taylor, R., Van Buyten, J., & Buchser, E. (2005). Spinal cord stimulation for chronic back and leg pain and failed back surgery syndrome: A systematic review and analysis of prognostic factors. *Spine*, 30, 152–160.

Townsend C, Rome J, Bruce B, et al. (2011). Chapter 8: Interdisciplinary pain rehabilitation programs. In Ebert M, Kerns R (eds). *Behavioral and Pharmacological Pain Management*. Cambridge University Press: New York, NY.

Turk, D., Wilson, H., & Cahana, A. (2011). Treatment of chronic non-cancer pain. *Lancet*, 377, 2226–2235.

Turner, J., Loeser, J., Deyo, R., & Sanders, S. (2004). Spinal cord stimulation for patients with failed back surgery syndrome or complex regional pain syndrome: A systematic review of effectiveness and complications. *Pain*, 108, 137–147.

Turner, J., Sears, J., & Loeser, J. (2007). Programmable intrathecal opioid delivery systems for chronic noncancer pain: A systematic review of effectiveness and complications. *Clinical Journal of Pain*, 23, 180–195.

Tyson R, Strong J. (1990). Adaptive equipment: Its effectiveness for people with chronic lower back pain. *OTJR: Occupation, Participation and Health*, 10, 111–121.

US Department of the Army, Office of the Surgeon General. (2010) Pain Management Task Force Final Report. Available at: http://www.regenesisbio.com/pdfs/journal/Pain_Management_Task_Force_Report.pdf. Accessed September 28, 2015.

van Tulder, M., Malmivaara, A., Hayden, J., & Koes, B. (2007). Statistical significance versus clinical importance: Trials on exercise therapy for chronic low back pain as example. *Spine*, 32, 1785–1790.

Webster LR, Choi Y, Desai H, Webster L, Grant BJ. Sleep-disordered breathing and chronic opioid therapy. *Pain Med*. 2008; 9:425–32.

Wielandt T, Strong J. (2000). Compliance with prescribed adaptive equipment: A literature review. *British Journal of Occupational Therapy*, 63, 65–75.

Young, R., Kroening, R., Fulton, W., et al. (1985). Electrical stimulation of the brain in treatment of chronic pain: Experience over 5 years. *Journal of Neurosurgery*, 62, 389–396.

Chapter 4

Psychological Interventions

Past research has found that psychological treatment, as a whole, results in modest improvements in pain and physical and emotional functioning. Psychological interventions include

- behavioral therapy
- cognitive-behavioral therapy
- psychodynamic therapy
- stress management
- emotional disclosure
- biofeedback
- hypnosis

There is insufficient evidence to recommend one therapeutic approach over another. Psychological interventions aim to

- modify the overall pain experience
- help restore functioning
- improve the quality of life of people who suffer from chronic pain

The modest reductions in pain witnessed with psychological interventions are similar to those noted with traditional approaches.

Questions for the Reader to Ponder

By the end of this chapter, you should be able to answer the following questions:

1. Is mindfulness a form of relaxation technique?
2. What biological signals are measured during biofeedback?
3. What is cognitive-behavioral therapy?
4. How does it feel to be hypnotized?

The field of psychotherapy has witnessed several ways of thinking over time, or "waves." The first wave was psychoanalysis, emphasizing on the unconscious conflicts, early experiences, and transference. The second wave was behavior modification, stemming from learning theories. The second wave was organized into procedures for desensitization and changing contingences. The third wave was humanistic/experiential psychotherapy, emphasizing emotions, conscious motives, and human potential. The fourth wave is cognitive psychotherapy, emphasizing on thoughts and interpretations. The most recent wave is considered the mindfulness-based therapies, which incorporate meditation practices.

A Closer Look
What are different types of meditation?

Meditation involves several techniques, including compassion, love, patience, and mindfulness. Mindfulness is a type of meditation. There are other practices which fall under meditation.

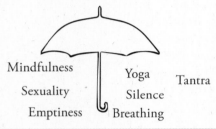

Mindfulness
Sexuality
Emptiness
Yoga
Silence
Breathing
Tantra

Meditation

Meditation is a devotional exercise of or leading to observation. Practicing short meditation exercises is a great way to break away from pain. It may also reduce anxiety, depression, and sleep trouble. Meditation is an umbrella term that encompasses the practices of

- reaching ultimate consciousness and concentration
- acknowledging the mind and regulating attention

Mindfulness is not some special mystical state, nor is it a form of relaxation. Mindfulness is an exercise in just noticing or being aware. There are several types of mindfulness-based interventions available, including

- Mindfulness-Based Stress Reduction (MBSR)
- Mindfulness-Based Cognitive Therapy (MBCT)
- Dialectical behavior therapy (DBT)
- Acceptance & Commitment Therapy (ACT)

MBSR uses a combination of mindfulness meditation, body awareness, and yoga to help people become more mindful. MBCT uses traditional cognitive-behavioral therapy methods and adds in mindfulness meditation. DBT combines standard cognitive-behavioral techniques for emotion regulation with concepts of distress tolerance. DBT is derived from Buddhist meditative practice and uses mindfulness as a core exercise. ACT is a form of clinical behavior analysis that uses acceptance and mindfulness strategies. It is mixed with commitment and behavior-change strategies to increase psychological flexibility. ACT will be the only one discussed in more detail because it has been shown to have strong research support for the treatment of chronic pain.

A Closer Look

How do I practice mindful meditation at home?

1. Find a quiet place to practice where there are few distractions
2. Commit to a set amount of time—turn off your phone and let others know
3. Sit in a comfortable position—close your eyes but make sure you remain alert
4. Notice the position of your body and any sensations
5. Notice your breathing—breathe slowly and naturally
6. Notice if your mind wanders—your mind will wander but don't judge
7. Assume a passive attitude—let go of any worries about doing this right
8. The purpose is not to stop the mind from wandering but just to notice where it wanders
9. Continue for 10 to 20 minutes—try to glance at a clock rather than setting a timer
10. At the end of the exercise sit comfortably for 1 or 2 minutes and stand slowly when you are ready

Acceptance & Commitment Therapy (ACT)

Acceptance & Commitment Therapy (ACT) is one of the more actively researched approaches among the "new" wave psychotherapies. It is a style of therapy with a lot of flexibility, and the therapeutic process is more experiential than didactic. Therefore, efficacy will depend largely on your level of commitment and participation in treatment. The experiential elements will challenge you to learn and practice new and more flexible ways of responding to pain. The basic idea of ACT is for you to shift your primary focus from reducing or eliminating pain to fully engaging in your life. ACT is about changing how you relate with your internal experiences. It is about living better! A primary goal of treatment is for you to suffer less through becoming actively involved in what you really care about. You will do what matters most in your life despite having and experiencing pain. ACT treatment is difficult, as there are no simple solutions to chronic pain.

Patients report feeling a range of emotions during the intervention, but this response is natural and incredibly human. The role of the therapist is to help you accept whatever discomfort exists, both physical and emotional. You learn to live with this while continuing to live your life according to your values. Doing so can help you to make meaningful changes in your life and reduce suffering. ACT applies six core treatment processes through different experiential exercises to create psychological flexibility. The model is best illustrated using a hexaflex. A simplified model may suggest the intervention helps you to become more open, be present, and take action.

The Acceptance & Commitment Therapy Hexaflex

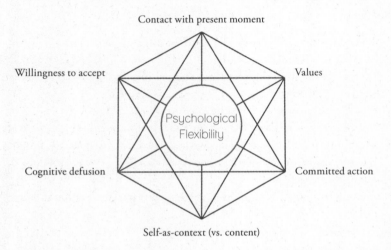

You will learn to become more "open" to your experience of pain using two principles, willingness to accept and cognitive defusion. The principle of willingness to accept describes the process of allowing internal experiences regarding pain to come and go. You experience thoughts, feelings, body sensations, and memories without struggling with or becoming fused with them. When learning about cognitive defusion, you begin to create distance from these experiences and perceive them as what they are. They are only thoughts, feelings, body sensations, and memories of pain! This can work to help you create distance from these experiences and realize that you are not identified by your thoughts. This way, you can work to respond to these experiences through evaluating their workability given your values rather than accepting or buying into them in a literal way.

A Closer Look

What do you mean, I have to accept my pain?

Acceptance does mean having to accept living with a certain amount of pain. Acceptance does not mean that you have to give up all hope and feel defeated. Acceptance does not mean that you have to accept someone else's version of your condition. Acceptance does not mean not caring. Healthy acceptance means recognizing that no amount of agonizing over and bemoaning your fate is going to make things any better.

True acceptance means coming to terms mentally and emotionally with your unpleasant reality.

Imagine that one day you decide to throw a party for all your friends. You call all your friends and tell them anyone can come. Days before the big event, you get your place ready for the party and are really excited to see everyone. Everyone you expected has RSVPed to your invitation for your party. But then you find out that someone you definitely did not want to come to your party is planning to go. It's your annoying neighbor Joe. Joe is rude and grumpy, moans a lot, acts a little weird, and has poor hygiene. He is definitely someone you don't want at your party.

You have a few choices in this situation.

1. Teach Joe to behave properly first, then have your party.
2. Numb yourself from reacting to Joe by using drugs or alcohol before the party starts.
3. Avoid Joe altogether by not having the party.
4. Plan to suppress your reactions to Joe by keeping yourself busy during the party.
5. Be willing to accept Joe just as he is, with his poor hygiene and his bad attitude, and still have your party.

Note: You cannot get rid of Joe. In this example, Joe is your pain. After reviewing all the options available, the only realistic option is #5. You must learn to accept your pain and move forward in your life.

You will learn to become more "present" with the experience of pain using two other principles, contact with the present moment and observing the self. The principle of making contact with the present moment describes how you become more aware of and experience the here and now. Mindfulness is essential to this process! The purpose is not to change or judge, but rather to be fully in the present moment, noticing when the mind wanders and bringing it back. It involves being able to operate from a different and separated point of view. The aim of mindfulness is to increase awareness of your body functions and feelings and the content of your thoughts. Each therapy session begins with a mindfulness exercise. Observing the self involves you accessing a transcendent sense of self, a continuity of consciousness which is always changing. In other words, you will learn to contact your thoughts and feelings about pain from the perspective of a separate observer.

A Closer Look

What do you mean the brain is not your friend?

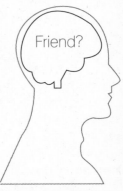

Imagine that a page from this book is a $100 bill. Would you want this piece of paper? Now imagine that I crumple this paper. Do you still want it? Now imagine that I stomp on the paper. Do you still want it? Now imagine that I tear the paper in half. Is it still something that you want? Most people say "yes" up to this point. Now imagine that I blow my nose in the paper. Do you still want it?

If your brain said "no," then it decided that the $100 was not worth it anymore because it is now "gross." But if your brain said yes, then congratulations are in order. You are now $100 richer. The point of this exercise is two-fold. First, a real $100 bill is nothing more than a piece of paper we all agreed is worth $100. Secondly, your brain is not always your friend. If you listened to your brain when it said "no," then you lost $100. This is why learning about cognitive defusion is important in ACT.

You will also learn to "take action" despite your experience of pain using two more principles, valued directions and committed action. The principle of valued directions describes the process of discovering what is most important to your true self, whether it be personal growth, leisure, citizenship, social relationships, health, work/education, spirituality, family, parenting, and/or intimate relationships. Making a committed action involves setting goals according to your values and carrying them out responsibly. You will be asked to state and write down commitments in the form of specific, meaningful, adaptive, realistic, and time-framed steps that you are willing to take in your valued directions along with what activities. At the end of the intervention, you will be taught how to maintain your progress by continuing to

1. practice mindfulness and acceptance exercises
2. set short-term goals each week
3. monitor your progress

You will also be prepared for relapse and setbacks. You will be able to identify when you have relapsed or had a setback on your chosen path. When you fail to live up to or keep your valued commitments, you be trained to recommit to your valued action plan. You then get back on track by noticing the setback and bringing your awareness back to your valued directions.

ACT and traditional cognitive-behavioral therapy (CBT) are among the most utilized interventions in behavioral medicine for pain. Past research has shown that ACT compares favorably with CBT in the treatment of chronic pain among different populations. They tend to overlap in terms of behavioral techniques and strategies. But there are specific theoretical differences that exist with regard to the role of cognitions and emotional regulation strategies. ACT has been shown to have modest support, but CBT has strong, longstanding research support to treat chronic, non-cancer pain according to the American Psychological Association.

A Closer Look
How do I make a committed action plan?

Step 1: Choose an area of life to work on.

Step 2: The underlying values of my goals in these domains are

_____.

- **Specific:** Be specific about what actions you are committed to taking.
- **Meaningful:** Notice if your intention is authentically guided by your values as opposed to a goal.
- **Adaptive:** Ask yourself if your goal is going to be moving you forward to enhance or improve your quality of life.
- **Realistic:** Find a balance between setting overly easy and unattainable goals.
- **Time-framed:** Get even more specific about your goal by setting a time and date by which you plan to accomplish it.

Step 3: My values-based goals are

- Short-term goal(s): List some things you can do in the service of your values-based goal within the next few days and weeks:

  _____.

- Long-term goal(s): Make a plan of what actions will move you closer to your values-based goal over the next few months and years:

  _____.

Biofeedback

The term biofeedback refers to the function of this modality. *Bio* means body and *feedback* is having information fed back to you. Biofeedback is the use of instruments to mirror psychological and physical processes an individual is not normally aware of and bring them under voluntary control. The fight or flight response involves all parts of the nervous system, including the sympathetic nervous system. The sympathetic nervous system is also responsible for adrenaline secretion. The response occurs when an individual is subjected to severe stress. When the response is activated by a stressor, the nervous system increases sympathetic activity. This includes an increased heart rate, sweating, and muscular strength, which prepares the individual to face or avoid the stressor. Most people who benefit from biofeedback have conditions that are made worse by stress, which makes internal processes become overactive.

The biofeedback instruments will give you immediate information about your own biological conditions, including

- brainwaves
- heart function
- breathing
- muscle tension
- temperature
- sweat

This feedback enables an individual to become an active participant in the process of health maintenance. Over time, these changes can endure without continued use of the instruments. Providers may recommend biofeedback for several reasons. Biofeedback training may be able to reduce, or even eliminate, the need for medication management of disease states. Biofeedback may also help you take an active role in your own healing, which is consistent with the self-management model of chronic pain.

Believe it or not, most individuals have come into contact with common types of biofeedback. For example, people use

- thermometers
- bathroom scales
- mirrors
- mood rings
- Fitbits

They use these at home to become more aware of their physiology. They use the information they obtain from these to make changes and gain control. People also come in contact with blood pressure and heart rate monitors when they are triaged into medical clinics, which provide information about their heart's functioning, which can be altered by stress. There are several types of instruments that are typically used in biofeedback training.

Thermistor: Perhaps the most common is the thermistor, a skin probe taped on a finger to measure temperature.

Photoplethysmograph: Also known as the heart rate variability (HRV) monitor, which involves taping a probe on the index finger. It detects the flushing of the skin that occurs with each heart contraction.

Pnuemograph: A sensor placed around your abdomen which measures breath rate, rhythm, volume, and location.

Electrodermograph: Another sensor that can be placed on the palm of the hand or the surface of the fingers which measures sweat.

Electromyograph (EMG): The most widely used of all biofeedback instruments. EMG monitors muscle tension, body relaxation, and muscle dysfunction. The sensors are attached to the area of tension, but the most basic placement for training is on the forehead.

Electroencephalograph (EEG): Also known as neurofeedback, it is likely the most complicated form of biofeedback. The EEG measures electrical activity in the brain using sensors on a scalp cap.

Biofeedback instruments do not change or influence bodily processes; they merely monitor or measure bodily functions. Implementing mental exercises is the key! In a typical biofeedback training session, sensors are attached to the skin at the different locations of the body. This, of course, is done only after the therapist has asked for your permission. The area of the skin where the sensor is going to be attached is usually cleaned with alcohol or a dab of electrode gel is applied to each sensor. The biofeedback therapist then leads you in mental exercises. These techniques can include

- listening to pre-recorded audio or other media
- practicing mindfulness
- engaging in formal relaxation techniques
- conducting prescribed self-hypnosis practice

When successful, the feedback signals from these instruments reflect accomplishment. The signals act as affirmation and encouragement for your continued efforts.

A Quick Biofeedback Guide

Modality	Measures
Thermistor	Peripheral blood flow, temperature
Photoplethysmograph	Peripheral blood flow, heart rate variability (HRV)
Pnuemograph	Abdominal/chest movement, respiration rate
Electrodermograph	Sweat gland activity
Electromyograph (EMG)	Muscle action potentials
Electroencephalograph (EEG)	Cortical postsynaptic potentials

There are three stages that occur during the biofeedback training:

Stage 1: You gain awareness of your problematic physical response. Individuals identify how their bodies respond to stressors and determine their ability to overcome the undesired physical reactions.

Stage 2: You use the signals from the biofeedback to control your physical responses. The individual is coached by the therapist to reach certain goals related to managing a specific physical response.

Stage 3: You transfer control from the biofeedback equipment to yourself. Individuals learn through trial and error to identify triggers that alert them to implement the self-regulation skills learned. You will be encouraged daily practice of the mental exercises at the conclusion of treatment.

Biofeedback should be conducted only by trained health care professionals, such as licensed psychologists or master's level clinicians. There are some contraindications for biofeedback that you must keep in mind. Certain cases are discouraged to pursue biofeedback therapy, including:

- persons with severe psychosis or neurosis
- individuals with a pacemaker or other implantable electrical device
- debilitated patients
- patients with psychopathic personalities

Biofeedback should only be used as an adjunct to, not a replacement treatment for depression, diabetes, and other endocrine disorders. Biofeedback is considered to be an otherwise safe, non-medication intervention that does not appear to have any negative side effects. A positive side effect of biofeedback is you can use self-regulation skills to help manage other life stressors. You can use these skills anywhere at any time independently from medications or doctors.

Relaxation Techniques

The biofeedback therapist may coach you and use relaxation techniques to help facilitate changes. The purpose of these exercises is to decrease autonomic nervous system activity, such as:

- oxygen consumption
- heart rate
- blood pressure
- muscle tension

Relaxation exercises have been found to be useful for pain caused by

- muscle tension
- arthritis
- procedural pain
- postoperative pain
- cancer pain
- cognitive and affective components of pain

There are several different types of relaxation exercises, including—but not limited to—diaphragmatic breathing, guided imagery, progressive muscle relaxation (PMR), and autogenics.

Diaphragmatic Breathing: the act of breathing deep into your lungs by flexing your diaphragm rather than breathing shallow from your rib cage. It is marked by expansion of the abdomen rather than the chest when breathing. It is generally considered a healthier and fuller way to ingest oxygen. It is often used as a therapy for pain management. Performing diaphragmatic breathing can be therapeutic, and with enough practice, can become a standard way of breathing. To breathe diaphragmatically, or with the diaphragm, you must draw air into lungs in a way which will expand stomach and not chest. It is best to perform these breaths as long, slow intakes of air. Allow the body to absorb all the inhaled oxygen while simultaneously relaxing the breath. To do this comfortably, it is often best to loosen tight-fitting clothes. Restrictive clothes can interfere with your body's ability to intake air. At first you may not feel comfortable expanding the stomach during diaphragmatic breathing. It actually fills up the majority of the lungs with oxygen, much more than chest-breathing or shallow breathing.

A Closer Look

How do I practice diaphragmatic breathing?

1. Sit or lie comfortably while wearing loose garments
2. Put one hand on your chest and one on your stomach
3. Slowly inhale through your nose or through pursed lips (to slow down the intake of breath)
4. As you inhale, feel your stomach expand with your hand
5. Slowly exhale through pursed lips to regulate the release of air
6. Rest and repeat

Guided Imagery: A therapeutic technique in which a facilitator uses descriptive language intended to psychologically benefit mental imagery. This often involves several or all the senses in the mind of the listener. The facilitator may precede the guided imagery with diaphragmatic breathing. Guided imagery is using your imagination to create sensory images that decrease your pain. It has been found to be useful for back pain, postoperative pain, arthritis pain, headache, and cancer pain. The length is tailored to your preference and energy level. Often, guided imagery sessions can use an audiotaped script or a live guide. Caution is given for this technique to be used in patients with dissociative disorders.

A Closer Look

How do I practice guided imagery? Here is an example:

1. Loosen your clothing, take off your shoes, and sit comfortably in a chair. Dim the lights, if you prefer. Close your eyes. Take in a few deep breaths. Picture yourself descending an imaginary staircase. With each step, notice that you feel more and more relaxed.

2. When you feel relaxed, imagine a favorite scene. It could be a beach, a mountain slope, or a particularly enjoyable moment with friends and family. Try to go into this scene each time you practice your imagery. If you can create a special, safe place where nothing can hurt you and you feel secure, it will make you more receptive to other images.

3. Once you feel comfortable in your favorite scene, gradually direct your mind toward the ailment you're concerned about. Let the image of the ailment become more vivid and in focus. Don't worry if it seems to fade in and out.

4. If several images come to mind, choose one and stick with it for that session. On the other hand, if no images come to mind, try focusing on a different sensation. For instance, imagine hearing bacon frying in a skillet or smelling wildflowers in a meadow. If all else fails, think about how you feel at the moment. Angry? Frustrated? What color is that anger? What image is evoked? Use these feelings to forge images.

5. Each time you do this exercise, imagine that your ailment is completely cured at the end of the session. Take a few more deep breaths and picture yourself re-climbing the imaginary staircase and gradually becoming aware of your surroundings. Open your eyes, stretch, smile, and go on with your day.

Progressive Muscle Relaxation (PMR): A technique for reducing anxiety by alternately tensing and relaxing muscles. PMR entails a physical and mental component. The physical component involves the tensing and relaxing of different muscle groups of the body. With the eyes closed, tension in a given muscle group is purposefully done for approximately 10 seconds and then released for 20 seconds. This is done before continuing with the next muscle group in the sequence. The mental component focuses on the difference between the feelings of the tension and relaxation. Because your eyes are closed, your concentration is focused on the sensation of tension and relaxation.

A Closer Look

How do I practice progressive muscle relaxation?
Here is an example:

1. Start by getting into a comfortable sitting position. Close your eyes. Place your feet flat on the floor, legs uncrossed and your hands resting comfortably at your side or on your lap.

2. Begin by noticing your breathing, noticing your abdomen rise and fall with each breath (pause after each breath). As your breathing becomes more relaxed and restful, take your awareness up to your face. Then you'll start this process with the muscles in your face.

3. Tense the muscles in the face by making a sour face, like you ate a lemon, hold that face for four seconds, and then release the muscles in your face. Repeat the process two times.

4. Notice the tension just washing away. With each tense and release cycle, you'll notice it becomes easier and easier to release and relax each muscle group. Repeat the process of tensing muscles, except you should be inhaling through the nose and exhaling through the mouth, relaxing even more with each breath.

5. Now, you should move your awareness to the shoulder and neck area. Notice the muscles in the shoulder and neck area. Tense the muscles in the neck by pressing the shoulders towards the ears and holding for a count of four seconds and then release. With your awareness in the neck and shoulders, now tense them and hold for four seconds and release.

6. Bring your awareness to the muscles in the arms. Tense the muscles in both of your arms by curling the arms up towards your biceps and holding them as if you are lifting weights and holding them to your chest, holding for four seconds and then release.

7. Now, bring your awareness to the muscles in the hands. Tense the muscles in the hands by clenching it into a tight fist, holding for a count of ten seconds and then release. With your awareness in the hands, now tense the muscles in your hands and hold for four seconds and release.

8. Notice the muscles in the upper back, around the shoulder blades. Tense the muscles in the upper back by pressing the shoulder blades together and holding for a count of four seconds and then release. With your awareness in the shoulder blades, now tense and hold for four seconds, and release.

9. Now, notice the muscles in the abdomen and low back. Tense the muscles in the abdomen by imaging that you are trying to touch the belly button to the spine, pressing the low back to the chair and holding for a count of four

seconds and then release. With your awareness in the abdomen, now tense and hold for four seconds, and release.

10. Now, notice the muscles in your thighs. Tense the muscles in the thighs by raising one leg at a time for ten seconds. Keep your back against the chair. You can use your arms to hold yourself down into the chair.

11. Now on the feet. Tense these muscles by pointing the toes towards the knees, and again holding for three seconds, and then releasing the calf muscles. With your awareness in the calf muscles, now tense the calves and hold for four seconds, and release.

Autogenic Training: This exercise involves repeating a set of visualizations that induce a state of relaxation. Autogenic training engages mind and body in deep relaxation, reversing the stress response. The resulting altered state of consciousness allows spontaneous, often subtle, psychological and physiological changes. This is a unique experience for each person. Autogenic means self-generated or self-regulated and teaches your body to respond to your commands. You will learn to gain control over body functions that you normally have no control over, such as heart rate, blood pressure, digestion, body temperature, and breathing. Autogenic training can help you with many kinds of physical and mental health conditions, including migraines, pain disorders, Raynaud's disease, sleep disorders, and tension headaches. Relaxation is only one of the techniques that you will learn if you are treated with cognitive-behavioral therapy.

A Closer Look

How do I practice autogenics? Here is an example:

1. Sit in the meditative posture and mentally scan the body.

2. Repeat each of the following sentences three times. Breathe deeply, one count in, one count out, and silently repeat the following formula—the first half of the phrase (the part before the "/") as you inhale, the second half (the part after the "/") as you exhale:

   "my right arm/is heavy"
   "my arms and legs/are heavy and warm"
   "my heartbeat/is calm and regular"
   "my body/breathes freely and easily"
   "my abdomen/is warm"
   "my forehead/is cool"
   "my neck and shoulders/are heavy"
   "my mind/is quiet and still"
   "I am/at peace"

3. Slowly repeat these phrases only once:

"Each time I practice these exercises, I gain more of my desires."

"Every day, in every way, I am becoming healthier."

"Now as I prepare to return to my normal level of awareness, I see myself bringing with me . . . the health . . . happiness . . . comfort . . . and love that I feel and see. I take another deep relaxing breath, open my eyes, stretch comfortably, and see myself filled with heavy energy."

Cognitive-Behavioral Therapy (CBT)

I want you to do something before you continue reading about this modality. Please, go online on your phone or computer and type in the words "cognitive-behavioral therapy" and "chronic pain" in your search engine and see how many results come up. Cognitive-behavioral therapy (CBT) is perhaps the most investigated and research supported modality available for chronic pain. CBT is a structured, time-limited, present-focused approach to psychotherapy that helps you engage in an active coping process. This process is aimed at changing maladaptive thoughts and behaviors that can serve to maintain and exacerbate the experience of chronic pain. Past research has shown CBT to be highly successful in the treatment of different pain disorders, including

- fibromyalgia
- headaches
- low back pain
- osteoarthritic knee pain
- rheumatoid arthritis pain

CBT for pain is based upon the cognitive-behavioral model of pain. The cognitive-behavioral model is grounded on the notion that pain is a complex experience that is influenced by the individual's underlying cognitions, affect, and behavior. In other words, "As I think, so I feel (and do)!"

CBT for pain has three components: a treatment rationale, coping skills training, and the application and maintenance of learned coping skills. The goals of CBT are to

1. reduce the impact pain has on your daily life
2. learn skills for coping better with your pain
3. improve physical and emotional functioning
4. reduce pain and your reliance on pain medications

CBT protocols introduce cognitive concepts, such as automatic thinking and cognitive restructuring. Automatic thoughts spontaneously come to mind when a particular situation occurs. Cognitive distortions, unconscious operations of the mind, are categories of automatic thinking. People do not choose their cognitive distortions, but act on them without even being aware of their negative implications. Negative thinking opens the "gate" from the Gate Control Theory and causes an increase in pain perception. The first step to changing cognitive distortions is to recognize them. Negative cognitive distortions fall into four broad categories:

- overgeneralization (taking isolated cases and using them to make wide generalizations)
- mental filters (focusing on negative aspects of an event while ignoring positive aspects)
- jumping to conclusions (drawing decisions from little evidence)
- emotional reasoning (making decisions based on personal feeling rather than evidence)

Cognitive restructuring is a useful tool for understanding and turning around negative thinking. It involves observing negative thoughts closely, challenging them, and re-scripting the negative thinking that lies behind them. In engaging in this active process, you learn to approach situations in a positive frame of mind. The key idea behind cognitive restructuring is the A-B-C model, which purports that interpretations of the environment (or activating event: A) affect cognitions (or the beliefs about the event: B), which in turn drive our emotions and bodily sensations (or consequences: C).

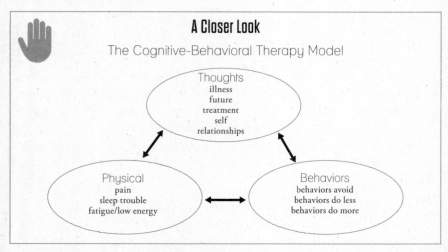

A Closer Look

The Cognitive-Behavioral Therapy Model

Thoughts
illness
future
treatment
self
relationships

Physical
pain
sleep trouble
fatigue/low energy

Behaviors
behaviors avoid
behaviors do less
behaviors do more

CBT protocols also introduce behavioral strategies, such as relaxation techniques, time-based activity pacing, and pleasant activity scheduling. There are several types of relaxation techniques employed in CBT, including diaphragmatic breathing, progressive muscle relaxation (PMR), and visual imagery.

A Closer Look
What is time-based activity pacing?

Time-based activity pacing instruction is a singular behavioral intervention to manage pain symptoms. Typically, people who suffer from chronic pain will engage in a lot of activity on their good day, and then they stay off their feet the next few days.

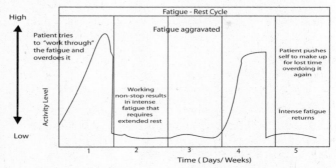

I like to call this the bunny ears phenomenon. This behavior is not therapeutic. Instead, we encourage people to engage in similar amounts of activity daily. The key is to stop the activity BEFORE you feel pain increasing. In order to do this, there are four steps to time-based pacing, or an activity-rest cycle:

1. List some things you tend to overdo
2. Limit the amount of time for the activity
3. Stop the activity and rest when the time is completed (not the task)
4. Repeat the cycle until the task is complete

This type of behavior is therapeutic and rehabilitative.

A Closer Look
What is pleasant activity scheduling?

Pleasant activity scheduling is another way to increase positive emotions and to "close" the gate. There are four steps to pleasant activity scheduling:

1. List activities that you think might be pleasurable
2. Rate each activity according to your current ability
3. Schedule the activities during the next week
4. Review progress and attempt again during the next month

Below is a list of activities that you can explore. Not all the activities are right for everyone:

- Shopping (window)
- Reading or writing
- Fishing, hunting, or camping
- Yard sales
- Spectator sports
- Going to church or praying
- Relaxation or yoga
- Exercise/sports
- Sex/affection
- Having visitors
- Group activities
- Dancing
- Yard work
- Mechanics
- Crafts (all types) or hobbies
- Cooking or eating out
- Going to the library/bookstore
- Music (play & listen), singing, art
- Walking (in/outdoors)
- Games/cards
- Travel
- Volunteer work
- Bubble bath or hot shower
- Making phone calls
- Sending mail or emailing a friend
- Taking care of pets/plants
- Watching TV/movies or listening to radio
- Smiling

At the end of the intervention, you will create a plan on how to use the skills learned when you have a pain flare-up. The plan involves four steps:

1. Prepare for a flare-up before it occurs
2. Confront the flare-up head-on (do not ignore it)
3. Avoid pitfalls during critical moments (watch out for cognitive distortions)
4. Reflect about what skills were successful and create a new plan for the next flare-up. There will be next time!

Hypnosis

Hypnosis is a procedure involving cognitive processes like imagination in which you are guided by a health professional to respond to suggestions. These suggestions are for changes in perceptions, sensations, thoughts, feelings, and behaviors. According to the Society of Psychological Hypnosis (Division 30), hypnosis involves learning how to use your mind and thoughts in order to manage

- emotional distress
- unpleasant physical symptoms
- certain habits or behaviors

Sometimes, people are also trained in self-hypnosis, in which they learn to guide themselves through a hypnotic procedure. There are many myths, misconceptions, and misinformation about hypnosis. The number of misconceptions is much more than any other treatment for chronic pain! This is most likely due to the privileged position that hypnosis holds in popular culture via movies (*Get Out*, *Office Space*, *Shallow Hal*, *Zoolander*), books (*The Manchurian Candidate*), television (*Doctor Who*; *Monk*), rumors, and stage performers that make no attempt to tell the truth about hypnosis. These types of cultural references to hypnosis tend to embellish in order to make a more dramatic affect for entertainment purposes. In addition, medical hypnosis is not generally taught as part of a proper medical or health provider curriculum. This lack of knowledge adds to superstition even in the medical community. Clinical hypnosis should be conducted only by trained health care professionals, such as licensed psychologists or master's level clinicians. You should provide informed consent before beginning the hypnotic process.

Health professionals who conduct hypnosis may not be comfortable providing this type of therapy to all patients. It is important to remember that the working relationship can have an effect on treatment outcomes. The current evidence suggests that hypnosis is increasing in popularity as a modality of interest in the treatment of chronic, non-cancer pain, specifically

- chronic pelvic pain
- fibromyalgia
- headaches
- irritable bowel syndrome
- gastrointestinal conditions
- lower back pain
- multiple sclerosis
- temporomandibular pain

A Closer Look

What are some of the myths and misconceptions about hypnosis?

Myth #1: The hypnotherapist can make you do things against your will.
  Truth: The hypnotherapist does not have power over you and cannot make you do anything against your will.

Myth #2: You can get stuck in hypnosis and never come out.
  Truth: If the hypnotherapist left the room and never returned, you would wake up when you noticed they stopped speaking or after a short nap.

Myth #3: When hypnotized, you are in a trance and have no control.
  Truth: When hypnotized, your body is very relaxed and your mind is focused and open to suggestion.

Myth #4: Everyone can be hypnotized.
  Truth: People differ in the degree to which they respond to hypnosis. The key to becoming hypnotized is the extent to which a person wants to be.

Myth #5: Hypnosis can cure anything or solve any personal problem.
  Truth: Hypnosis is a natural tool we all have available to us to help improve our lives in many great ways.

Myth #6: Only weak-minded people can be hypnotized.
  Truth: The contrary is true. It is easier to hypnotize people who are intelligent.

Myth #7: Deep hypnosis is necessary for good results.

    Truth: Any level of hypnosis from light to deep can bring good results

Myth #8: Hypnosis is dangerous.

    Truth: Hypnosis is safe and has few, if any, side effects. There are cases where it may be contraindicated.

Even though hypnosis will rarely provide a cure for chronic, non-cancer pain, it will help you self-regulate and influence your pain perception. At its most basic, hypnosis treatment consists of four stages:

- an "induction" (usually to focus your attention)
- a deepening (usually to deepen your relaxation of the body)
- suggestions (usually for changes in the client's experience of pain)
- debriefing (ending)

A Closer Look

How do I practice self-hypnosis? Here is an example:

1. Go to a quiet room and sit in any comfortable chair or couch. Do not cross your legs or any part of your body.
2. Make sure you are not going to be disturbed for at least half an hour.
3. Close your eyes and work to rid your mind of any feelings of fear, stress, or anxiety. When you begin, you might find it difficult not to think. You may find that thoughts keep intruding. When this happens, observe them and then let them slip away.
4. Recognize the tension in your body. Beginning with your toes, imagine the tension slowly falling away from your body and vanishing. Imagine it freeing each body part one at a time (starting with your toes and working its way up your body). Visualize each part of your body becoming lighter and lighter as the tension is removed.
5. Take slow, deep breaths. When you exhale, see the tension and negativity leaving in a dark cloud. As you inhale, see the air returning as a bright force filled with life and energy.
6. Appreciate the fact that you are now extremely relaxed. Imagine you are at the top of a flight of ten stairs which at the fifth step start to submerge into a pool of water. Tell yourself that you are going to descend the stairs, counting each step down, starting at ten. Picture each number in your mind. Imagine that each number you count is further down and one step closer to the bottom.
7. After each number, you will feel yourself drifting further and further into deep relaxation. Once you are at the fifth step imagine and truly feel the refreshing coolness of the water and tell yourself that you are stepping into

an oasis of purity and cleanliness. As you begin to descend the last five steps, start to feel the water getting higher and higher up your body. You should now start to feel somewhat numb and your heart will start to race a bit, but notice it and let any worries about the situation just drift away into the water.

8. At this point at the bottom of the stairs, you shouldn't really feel anything, just a floating sensation. You may even feel like you're spinning. Once you have achieved this state you should proceed to address your problems and decide upon what it is you want from where you are.

9. Now start to narrate what you are doing, speak in the present and future tense quietly to yourself, or as if you are reading it from a page. You should avoid using statements with negative connotation such as "I don't want to be tired and irritable." Instead, say, "I am becoming calm and relaxed." Examples of positive statements if you have pain include "My back is beginning to feel wonderful."

10. Repeat your statement(s) to yourself as many times as you wish. Two or three times should be enough.

11. Once you are satisfied with what you have done and embraced, swim back to the stairs and feel, with each step you take, the water becoming lower and lower until you have once again reached that top step.

12. Once you have ascended, give yourself a few moments before opening your eyes. You may want to visualize yourself opening a door to the outside world. Do this slowly and imagine the light that pours in through the doorway; this should make your eyes open. Take your time getting up.

Beyond this basic structure, there are several variations in features of its practice. For example, if you used hypnosis for chronic pain, you could focus on changing the sensations from pain to something else or change focus of attention away from the pain. Sometimes underlying dynamics, motivations, or unresolved feelings may influence pain. Hypnosis can aid in this unconscious exploration and contribute to resolution. Additionally, individuals may be instructed to practice self-hypnosis outside of the treatment setting or may be provided audio recordings of the sessions to help assist with home practice.

Everyone responds to hypnosis differently. Some patients report their experience as a "trance-like" state. Others may experience it as imagery or the soothing of body sensations. Most people describe hypnosis as a pleasant experience and feel focused and absorbed in the experience, more alert, relaxed and comfortable, and peaceful. No matter what the experience, patients consistently report better health and happiness using these techniques. Imaging data has indicated that hypnosis affects cognitive control by modulating activity in specific brain areas. Hypnotized subjects have shown reduced brain activity in both visual areas and the anterior cingulate cortex, which plays a role in a wide variety of autonomic and cognitive functions. Certain cases are discouraged to pursue hypnosis, including anyone with severe psychological disorders that have gone untreated, persons under the influence of recreational drugs or alcohol, and anyone who is delusional or hallucinatory at the time of treatment. Some patients may object to hypnosis due to their religious beliefs, cultural beliefs, or external factors.

A Patient Story

A 58-year-old female goes to the pain clinic diagnosed with pseudogout and fibromyalgia in a wheelchair and cast on her right knee. She notes that she "hurt her knee so people would pay attention" (to her verbal complaints). She completes a course of treatment including cognitive-behavioral therapy for pain and acceptance and commitment therapy, and seems to be coping with her pain better. Every time she sees her provider, she exclaims, "there is my favorite doctor" and goes in for a hug.

 Was it the psychotherapy alone that accounts for the outcome or are there other factors to consider in this outcome? The answers are discussed in chapter 7.

Summary of the Research

Psychological interventions as a whole result in modest improvements in pain and physical and emotional functioning. There is insufficient evidence to recommend one therapeutic approach over another. Psychological interventions include

- behavioral therapy
- cognitive-behavioral therapy
- psychodynamic therapy
- emotional disclosure
- biofeedback
- hypnosis

Interestingly, the modest reductions in pain severity witnessed with psychological interventions were similar to those noted with traditional approaches.

Conclusion

In chapter 4, I reviewed the psychological approaches to chronic pain management, including meditation, acceptance and commitment therapy, biofeedback, relaxation techniques, cognitive-behavioral therapy, and hypnosis. Chapter 5 will review a group of modalities referred to as complementary and integrative health (CIH). These modalities include exercise and movement therapies, herbs and aromatherapy, spinal manipulation, traditional Chinese medicine, acupuncture, and healing touch.

References

American Psychological Association (APA). Hypnosis for the relief and control of pain. 2004. Available at: http://www.apa.org/research/action/hypnosis.aspx. Accessed: March 11, 2015.

APA Division 12. (2012). Psychological treatment of chronic or persistent pain. [Society of Clinical Psychology]. Available at: http://www.psychologicaltreatments.org. Accessed September 4, 2012.

Babu A, Mathew E, Danda D, et al. Management of patients with fibromyalgia using biofeedback: A randomized control trial. *Indian J Med Sci.* 2007; 61(8):455–461.

Barber T. Toward a theory of pain: Relief of chronic pain by prefrontal leucotomy, opiates, placebos, and hypnosis. *Psychol Bull.* 1959; 56:430–460.

Bastarache R, Bastarache R. *Hypotherapy certification training manual from A-Z.* Certified by the: American International Association of Hypnosis, 2005.

Boothby J, Thorn B, Stroud M, et al. (1999). *Coping with pain.* In R. Gatchel & D. Turk (Eds.). *Psychosocial factors in pain: Critical perspectives* (p. 343–359). New York, NY: Guilford Press.

Bordin E. The generalizability of the psychoanalytic concept of the working alliance. *Psychother Theory Res Pract.* 1979; 16: 252–260.

Bradley L, Young L, Anderson J, et al. (1987). Effects of psychological therapy on pain behavior of rheumatoid arthritis patients: Treatment outcome and six-month follow-up. *Arthritis & Rheumatism, 30,* 1105–1114.

Branstetter A, Wislon K, Hildebrandt M, et al. (2004). Improving psychological adjustment among cancer patients: ACT and CBT. Paper presented at the meeting of the Association for Advancement of Behavior Therapy, New Orleans.

Brown C, Barner J, Richards K, et al. Patterns of complementary and alternative medicine use in African Americans. *J Altern Complement Med.* 2007; 13(7):751–758.

Castel A, Perez M, Sala J, et al. Effect of hypnotic suggestion on fibromyalgic pain: Comparison between hypnosis and relaxation. *Eur J Pain.* 2007; 11(4):463–468.

Coulter I, Favreau J, Hardy M, et al. Biofeedback interventions for gastrointestinal conditions: A systematic review. *Altern Ther Health Med.* 2002; 8 (3):76–83.

Crider A, Glaros A, Gevirtz R, et al. Efficacy of biofeedback-based treatments for temporomandibular disorders. *Appl Psychophysiol Biofeedback.* 2005; 30 (4): 333–345.

Dahl J, Lundgren, T. (2006). *Living beyond your pain: Using acceptance & commitment therapy to ease chronic pain.* New Harbinger Publications.

Dahl J, Wilson K, Luciano C, et al. (2005). *Acceptance and commitment therapy for chronic pain.* Reno, NV: Context Press.

Duigan N, Burke A. (Unpublished Results). Group based treatment for chronic pain: Is ACT effective and how does it compare to CBT? Poster session presented at ACBS (Association for Contextual Behavioral Science), 4th Australian and New Zealand Conference, October 1–3, 2010, Adelaide, Australia.

Erickson M. Hypnosis in painful terminal illness. *J Ark Med Soc.* 1959; 56(2): 67–71.

Flaxman P, Bond F. (In Press). *Acceptance and commitment therapy in the workplace.* Chapter in Baer, R., (Ed.) *Mindfulness-based treatment approaches.* Elsevier.

Flor H, Birbaumer N. Comparison of the efficacy of electromyographic biofeedback, cognitive–behavioral therapy, and conservative medical interventions in the treatment of chronic musculoskeletal pain. *J Consult Clin Psychol.* 1993; 61(4): 653–658.

Forman E, Herbert J, Moitra E, et al. (2007). A randomized controlled effectiveness trial of acceptance and commitment therapy and cognitive therapy for anxiety and depression. *Behavior Modification, 31,* 772–799.

Glick R, Greco C. Biofeedback and primary care. *Prim Care Clin Office Pract.* 2010; 37 (2010) 91–103.

Goldenberg D, Kaplan K, Nadeau M, et al. (1994). A controlled study of a stress-reduction, cognitive-behavioral treatment program in fibromyalgia. *Journal of Musculoskeletal Pain, 2,* 53–66.

Hassett A, Radvanski D, Vaschillo E, et al. A pilot study of the efficacy of heart rate variability (HRV) biofeedback in patients with fibromyalgia. *Appl Psychophysiol Biofeedback.* 2007; 32 (1):1–10.

Hayes S, Strosahl K, Wilson K. (1999). *Acceptance and commitment therapy: An experiential approach to behavior change.* New York: Guilford Press.

Hoffman B, Papas R, Chatkoff D, et al. (2007). Meta-analysis of psychological interventions for chronic low back pain. *Health Psychology, 26,* 1–9.

Holroyd K, Nash J, Pingel J, et al. (1991). A comparison of pharmacological and nonpharmacological therapies for chronic tension headache. *Journal of Consulting and Clinical Psychology*, 59, 387–393.

Huet A, Lucas-Polomeni M, Robert J, et al. Hypnosis and dental anesthesia in children: A prospective controlled study. *Int J Clin Exp Hypnosis*. 2011; 59 (4): 424–441.

Jensen M, Barber J, Romano J, et al. A comparison of self-hypnosis versus progressive muscle relaxation in patients with multiple sclerosis and chronic pain. *Int J Clin Exp Hypnosis*. 2009; 57(2):198–221.

Jensen M, Ehde D, Gertz K, et al. Effect of self-hypnosis training and cognitive restructuring on daily pain intensity and catastrophizing in individuals with multiple sclerosis and chronic pain. *Int J Clin Exp Hypnosis*. 2011; 59 (1): 45–64.

Jensen M, Nielson W, Kerns R. (2003). Toward the development of a motivational model of pain self-management. *Journal of Pain*, 4, 477–492.

Jensen M. Hypnosis for chronic pain management: A new hope. *Pain*. 2009; 146 (3): 235–237.

Johnston M., Foster M., Shennan J., et al. (2010). The effectiveness of an acceptance and commitment therapy self-help intervention for chronic pain. *Clinical Journal of Pain*, 26, 393–402.

Keefe F, Caldwell D, Williams D, et al. (1990). Pain coping skills training in the management of osteoarthritic knee pain: A comparative study. *Behavior Therapy*, 21, 49–62.

Keefe F, Gil K. (1986). Behavioral concepts in the analysis of chronic pain syndromes. *Journal of Consulting and Clinical Psychology*, 54, 776–783.

Keefe F. (1996). Cognitive behavioral therapy for managing pain. *The Clinical Psychologist*, 49, 4–5.

Lamb S, Hansen Z, Lall R, et al. (2010). Group cognitive behavioral treatment for low-back pain in primary care: A randomized controlled trial and cost-effectiveness analysis. *Lancet*, 375, 916–923.

Lang E, Benotsch E, Fick L, et al. Adjunctive non-pharmacological analgesia for invasive medical procedures: A randomized trial. *Lancet*. 2000; 355 (9214): 1486–1494.

Lew M, Kravits K, Garberoglio C, et al. Uses of preoperative hypnosis to reduce postoperative pain and anesthesia-related side effects. *Int J Clin Exp Hypnosis*. 2011; 59 (4): 406–424.

Llewellyn Encyclopedia. Hypnosis myths. Available at: http://www.llewellynencyclopedia.com/print.php?what=article&id=222. Accessed: February 26, 2007.

McCracken L, Turk D. (2002). Behavioral and cognitive-behavioral treatment for chronic pain: Outcome, predictors of outcome, and treatment process. *Spine*, 27, 2564–2573.

McCracken L, Vowles K, Eccleston C. (2005). Acceptance-based treatment for persons with complex, long-standing chronic pain: A preliminary analysis of treatment outcome in comparison to a waiting phase. *Behavior Research and Therapy*, 43, 1335–1346.

McKay E, Kaufman R, Doctor U, et al. Treating vulvar vestibulitis with electromyographic biofeedback of pelvic floor musculature. *J Reprod Med*. 2001; 46 (4): 337–342.

Morley S, Eccleston C, Williams A. (1999) Systematic review and meta-analysis of randomized controlled trials of cognitive behavior therapy and behavior therapy for chronic pain in adults, excluding headache. *Pain*, 80, 1–13.

Nestoriuc Y, Martin A, Nestoriuc Y, et al. Efficacy of biofeedback for migraine: A meta-analysis. *Pain*. 2007; 128 (1-2) :111–127.

Nusbaum F, Redouté J, le Bars D, et al. Chronic low-back pain modulation is enhanced by hypnotic analgesic suggestion by recruiting an emotional network: A PET imaging study. *Int J Clin Exp Hypnosis*. 2011; 59 (1): 27–45.

Otis, J. (2007). *Managing Chronic Pain: A Cognitive-Behavioral Therapy Approach Therapist Guide (Treatments That Work)*. Oxford University Press, USA.

Picard P, Jusseaume C, Boutet M. Hypnosis for management of fibromyalgia. *Int J Clin Exp Hypnosis*. 2013; 61(1): 111–123.

Powers M, Vording M, Emmelkamp P. (2009). Acceptance and commitment therapy: A meta-analytic review. *Psychotherapy & Psychosomatics*, 78, 73–80.

Rainville P, Carrier B, Hofbauer R, et al. Dissociation of sensory and affective dimensions of pain using hypnotic modulation. *Pain*. 1999; 82 (2): 159–171.

Rainville P, Duncan G, Price D, et al. Pain affect encoded in human anterior cingulate but not somatosensory cortex. *Science*. 1997; 277(5328): 968–71.

Reid M, Otis J, Barry L, et al. (2003). Cognitive-behavioral therapy for chronic low back pain in older persons: A preliminary study. *Pain Medicine*, 4, 223–230.

Roberts L, Wilson S, Singh S, et al. Gut-directed hypnotherapy for irritable bowel syndrome: Piloting a primary care-based randomized controlled trial. *Br J Gen Pract*. 2006; 56(523):115–121.

Schwartz M, Andrasik F. *Biofeedback: A practitioner's guide (Third edition)*. Guilford Press; 2005.

Schwartz M. *Biofeedback: A practitioner's guide*. 3rd edition. New York: Guilford Press; 2003.

Simren M., Ringstrom G., Bjornsson E., Abrahamsson H. Treatment with hypnotherapy reducesthe sensory and motor component of the gastrocolonic response in irritable bowel syndrome. *Psychosom Med*. 2004; 66(2):233–238.

Spinhoven P., Linssen A., Van Dyck R., Zitman F. Autogenic training and self-hypnosis in the control of tension headache. *Gen Hosp Psychiatry.* 1992; 14(6):408–415.

Turk D., Meichenbaum D., Genest M. (1983). *Pain and behavioral medicine: A cognitive-behavioral perspective.* New York: Guilford Press.

Turner J, Clancy S. (1988). Comparison of operant-behavioral and cognitive-behavioral group treatment for chronic low back pain. *Journal of Consulting and Clinical Psychology, 58,* 573–579.

Veehof M, Oskam M, Schreurs K, et al. (2011). Acceptance-based interventions for the treatment of chronic pain: a systematic review and meta-analysis. *Pain, 152,* 533–542.

Vowles K, McCracken L. (2008). Acceptance and values-based action in chronic pain: A study of treatment effectiveness and process. *Journal of Consulting and Clinical Psychology, 76,* 397–407.

Vowles K, Sorrell J. (2007). *Life with chronic pain: An acceptance-based approach (Therapist guide and patient workbook).* School for Health, University of Bath: Centre for Pain Research.

Vowles K, Wetherell J, Sorrell J. (2009). Targeting acceptance, mindfulness, and values-based action in chronic pain: Findings of two preliminary trials of an outpatient group-based intervention. *Cognitive and Behavioral Practice, 16,* 49–58.

Wetherell J, Afari N, Rutledge T, et al. (2011). A randomized, controlled trial of acceptance and commitment therapy and cognitive-behavioral therapy for chronic pain. *Pain, 152,* 2098–2107.

Wicksell R, Melin L, Lekander M, et al. (2009). Evaluating the effectiveness of exposure and acceptance strategies to improve functioning and quality of life in longstanding pediatric pain: A randomized controlled trial. *Pain, 141,* 248–257.

Willmarth E, Willmarth K. *Biofeedback and hypnosis in pain management.* 2005.

Chapter 5

Complementary & Integrative Health Approaches

Complementary and integrative health (CIH), formerly known as complementary and alternative medicine (CAM), is a group of medical and healthcare systems and practices. It is estimated that more than one-third of adults use CIH in a given year. The top five reasons adults used CIH approaches are to treat back pain, neck pain, joint pain, arthritis, and other musculoskeletal conditions. CIH products can be categorized into four general categories:

- mind-body medicine (biofeedback, hypnosis, and exercise/yoga/ movement therapies)
- natural-biological based (aromatherapy and herbs)
- manipulation-body based (chiropractor, massage, and spinal manipulation)
- energy medicine (acupuncture and healing touch)

Questions for the Reader to Ponder

By the end of this chapter, you should be able to answer the following questions:

1. What are the goals of manipulation-body based therapies?
2. How does energy medicine work?
3. What are the modern methods used in Traditional Chinese Medicine?
4. What is healing touch?

I already reviewed some treatments in the previous chapter that are considered mind-body modalities, such as biofeedback and hypnosis. I want to spend some time discussing different types of movement programs that have shown to be successful for chronic pain.

Exercise & Movement Therapies

Physical exercise, or movement, is any bodily activity that enhances or maintains physical fitness and overall health and wellness. It is performed for various reasons, including:

- stretching
- strengthening
- aerobic/heart health
- simple enjoyment

Exercise is a successful treatment strategy in various conditions, including neck pain, osteoarthritis, headache, fibromyalgia, and low back pain.

Stretching, or flexibility exercises, can be good tools for managing chronic low back pain and fibromyalgia. There are several key points to stretching, including

1. Warm up before stretching.
2. Make slow, steady movements into a stretch—never bounce or jerk into a position.
3. Avoid locking joints in place—always have a very small amount of bend.

Other forms of flexibility exercises to consider are tai chi and yoga. Yoga has been known to help with arthritis, back and neck pain, headaches, and osteoporosis. When practicing yoga, regular benefits include improved sleep, strength and balance, circulation, flexibility, and physical and general well-being. There is promising scientific evidence to support the use of yoga and other movement-based exercises for non-cancer pain conditions, such as low back pain. These exercises may provide a good alternative when aerobic or strengthening exercises are not recommended.

Strengthening exercises work on muscles to help give added strength for strenuous activities. Strengthening exercises may help to manage chronic low back pain. There are some general guidelines for strengthening exercises, including

1. Avoid strengthening exercises of the same muscle group for two days in a row.
2. Gradually add weight to get the full benefit of the exercises.
3. Try to do 8 to 15 repetitions in a row.
4. Breathe out when lifting or pushing, and breath in to relax—avoid holding the breath.
5. Use smooth, steady movements—avoid jerking weights.
6. Avoid locking the arm and leg joints while exercising.

Aerobic (cardio) or heart health exercises can include walking, biking, and swimming and should be done regularly for a minimum of 30 minutes each. Here are some general guidelines for aerobic exercises:

1. Build stamina gradually, perhaps starting out with five minutes of activity at a time
2. Start out at a lower level of effort and work up gradually
3. Build up to at least 30 minutes of exercise on most days of the week
4. Exercise more often if not every day
5. Stretch before and after the activity when muscles are warm
6. Use safety equipment, like appropriate gym shoes, to prevent injuries

A typical fitness facility should be equipped with a variety of cardio, strength, and conditioning equipment.

Other Movement Therapies

Functional restoration is a rehabilitation program for chronic spine pain sufferers that aims to

- increase physical functioning
- improve pain-coping skills
- promote the return to a productive lifestyle at home/work
- limit the need for future spine treatments

At times, these programs can offer aquatic therapy. The unique physical properties of the water make it an ideal medium for rehabilitation for conditions, such as low back pain. A therapist will typically give constant attendance to the person receiving treatment in aquatic therapy.

Balneotherapy is the treatment of disease by bathing, usually practiced at spas. While it is considered distinct from hydrotherapy, there are some overlaps in practice and in underlying principles. Balneotherapy may involve hot or cold water, massage through moving water, relaxation, or stimulation. Many mineral waters at spas are rich in particular minerals such as silica, sulfur, selenium, radium, and medicinal clays.

Natural-Biological Based

The natural-biological based approaches have less research support available. Aromatherapy is a form of therapy that uses scents and essential oils from plant extracts to relieve the body of discomfort and pain. Different types of aromatherapy have been used throughout history across many cultures and countries to manage both acute and chronic pain for centuries. Most of the oils used in aromatherapy are strong, but you can use them at home.

A Quick Aromatherapy Guide

Essential Oil	Indications
Cedarwood	It has a soothing effect on the body and skin. It has a calming effect on the mind, and helps relieve anxiety and tension.
Chamomile	It has been known to help with tension, headaches, migraines, menstrual cramps, and back pain. It is also known to be a digestive aid.
Cinnamon	It promotes a healthy immune response and helps maintain a healthy lifestyle regimen. It provides a spicy and delicious addition when cooking.
Copaiba	It is from Brazil and has soothing properties. It is traditionally used to aid digestion and support the body's natural response to injury or irritation.
Cypress	It is refreshing and restores feelings of security and stability. It can be used to soothe sore muscles.
Frankincense	It has calming properties and can increase inner strength. It helps focus the mind and overcome stress and despair.
Ginger	It is commonly used to soothe, comfort, and balance digestive discomfort.
Lavender	It is touted as the best for pain management. It is helpful for muscle cramps and strains, headaches, neuralgia, and nervous tension, and it can help relieve mood swings.
Lemon	It is a source of d-limonene, which is known to support already healthy immune systems. It promotes energy and mental clarity.
Orange	It is added as a flavoring. It removes residue and negativity, increases conversation, and lifts depression.
Peppermint	It is used for restoring and soothing efficient digestion. It is uplifting and energizing and improves concentration and mental sharpness.
Sandalwood	It is considered to be one of the most valued for aromatherapy. It can soothe muscle tension, improve circulation, and help with sciatica.
Sweet Marjoram	It has potent sedative properties. It helps soothe muscle stiffness and cramps, improves circulation, and is used in treatment for rheumatism and osteoarthritis.
Vetiver	It helps detoxify tissue, balances the central nervous system, and can be beneficial for tension and depression.

Simply add a few drops in your bath water or use them as an aid for massage. Some diluted oils can also be delivered via the skin, smell, or orally with the consent of your physician. Most people who use aromatherapy do so as part of a whole-person approach to healthcare, not as a stand-alone treatment. With regard to regulation, the FDA classifies aromatherapy oils as a cosmetic, a drug, or both, depending on how the product is marketed.

Pain is multidimensional, and our tools for combating it should also reflect that. In terms of herbs, there are more than 100 plants known to have pain-relieving properties. You can access these herbs at your local health food store to fully restore your well-being. Research has shown that devil's claw, capsaicin from hot chiles, gamma-linolenic acid from seed oils, white willow, peppermint, and certain blended herbal extracts have medicinal properties.

A Quick Herb Guide

Herbal Extract	Indications
Arnica	It relieves osteoarthritic pain in knee and pain following carpal-tunnel release surgery. It is available in creams and tablets.
Boswellia	It can soothe pain from sports injuries and can help osteoarthritic knee pain.
Clove Oil	It is a popular home remedy for a toothache. Apply a drop or two of this excellent anti-inflammatory directly to your aching tooth or tooth cavity.
Capsaicin	It manipulates the body's pain status by hindering pain perception, triggering the release of pain-relieving endorphins and providing analgesic action. When using topical capsaicin products, be sure to avoid touching your eyes and other sensitive areas.
Devil's Claw	It eases muscular tension or pain in the back, shoulders, and neck. A popular treatment for osteoarthritic pain, it may ease rheumatoid arthritic pain as well. It is also available as tincture and tea. It should not be taken with blood-thinning medications.
Fennel	It is especially good for menstrual cramps. But avoid the herb while pregnant or nursing.
Feverfew	It is a remedy many people swear by for headaches, including migraines. Feverfew can reduce both the frequency and severity of headaches when taken regularly in capsules.
Gamma-Linolenic Acid (GLA)	It may help the body produce hormone-like substances that influence the immune system that can reduce inflammation. It curbs rheumatoid arthritic pain. It may also help with migraine headaches and mild diabetic nerve damage. Borage and black currant seed oils are the richest sources of GLA.
Gingerroot	It has analgesic and anti-inflammatory properties that can alleviate digestive cramps and mild pain from fibromyalgia.
Green Tea	It is great for stiff muscles—it has nine muscle-relaxing compounds, more than just about any other plant.

Licorice Root	It is recommended for sore throat. Do not take licorice if you have high blood pressure, heart conditions, diabetes, kidney disease, or glaucoma.
Oregano	Oregano, rosemary, and thyme are herbs you should be sprinkling liberally onto your food, as they are replete with analgesic, antispasmodic and anti-inflammatory compounds.
Peppermint	It is a famous antispasmodic for digestive cramps. Its antispasmodic and analgesic effects also can help relieve headaches, possibly including migraines, when applied to the forehead or temples as an oil.
White Willow	It is one of the oldest home analgesics for back, osteoarthritic, and nerve pains. Individuals with osteoarthritis of the knee or hip also are helped. It can be purchased as standardized extracts and teas. It may interact adversely with blood-thinning medications and other anti-inflammatory drugs.

Manipulation-Body Based

A resounding concept people with chronic non-cancer pain should embrace is that of "motion is lotion." It is the idea that a range of movement can improve or maintain function and promote health. It is also an idea rooted in the principles of several medical fields in which the movement of the body promotes health. These fields of medicine include

- osteopathic medicine
- chiropractic care
- allopathic care
- physical therapy
- massage therapy
- yoga

All of these forms of treatment are trying to promote motion. However, each is distinct in their own way.

In the United States there are two types of medical schools, the Doctor of Medicine (MD) and the Doctor of Osteopathic Medicine (DO) degrees. They are virtually indistinguishable, but most doctors hold the MD degree, while osteopaths hold the DO degree. The foremost principle for all doctors is to do no harm. The major difference between these types of doctors is that the DO practices by the osteopathic principles and has extra training in spinal manipulation.

The primary differences between a DO and other therapists are their levels of training and the scope of their practice. For example, a chiropractor is not an MD or DO. The chiropractor has their own Doctor of Chiropractic, or DC, and has not completed residency training in a hospital. The scope of chiropractic practice is defined by statute and is primarily concerned with normalizing the alignment of the spine to influence the relationship between the spinal column and the nervous system. The focus in DO treatment goes beyond simple spinal alignment by also addressing the abnormal body physiology using other techniques. There are four principles by which a DO approaches healthcare:

1. The human being is a dynamic unit of function
2. The body possesses self-regulatory mechanisms that are self-healing in nature
3. Structure and function are interrelated at all levels
4. Treatment is based on the understanding of the previous three principles

A DO applies these principles by striving to restore the body's normal structure and function, which promotes its self-healing nature. This means that the DO does not prescribe months or years of treatment at the first visit, but lets the prescription unfold as the treatment process proceeds. The National Center for Complementary & Integrative Health (NCCIH) still considers spinal manipulation by chiropractors as a CIH modality.

A Closer Look

How do manipulation-based providers differ in their training from traditional-based doctors?

Category	DO	MD	DC*
Undergrad training	4-year degree	Same	90 hours college credit; some require degree
Grad training	4-year DO degree	4-year MD degree	4-year DC degree
Post-grad training	1-year Internship 2–8 years Residency	Same	None
Licensure/Scope of practice	Fully licensed to practice the complete spectrum of medical and surgical specialties	Same	Licensed to practice chiropractic manipulation
Prescribe medications	Yes	Same	No
Manual medicine training	Over 500 hours	None	Over 500 hours

*According to the Association of Chiropractic Colleges and American Chiropractic Association

Massage therapists have their own certification, but are not doctors and have not completed residency training in a hospital. It is the position of the American Massage Therapy Association that massage can aid in pain relief. Research indicates that massage can reduce pain and pain intensity in people with metastatic bone pain, headache pain, postoperative pain, low back and leg pain, myalgia, cancer pain, carpal tunnel syndrome, and distal radial trauma.

Spinal Manipulation

Spinal manipulation is the practice of manual medicine to promote well-being. When structure is altered via the musculoskeletal system, abnormalities occur in other body systems. This can then produce restriction of motion, tenderness, tissue changes, and asymmetry. In other words, dysfunction in one area of the body is believed to derive from dysfunction from other areas of the body. Therefore, restoration of function in these areas might also help improve the symptoms and motion in area of concern. Some common problems treated by using spinal manipulation include mid-low back pain, neck pain, muscle tightness/stiffness, hip pain, fibromyalgia, muscle injury, scoliosis, some headaches, and muscle spasms. The goal of spinal manipulation is to improve the natural range of motion of the body by overcoming restrictions to normal motion. To do this, the provider will take a look at an extensive history with you and review any diagnostic tests that might help. The provider will also use their hands to palpate the body, looking for restrictions to normal range of motion while you remain clothed. The value of the placing of hands on the body is universally acknowledged by health professionals. This essential component of the doctor-patient relationship has a great deal to do with your well-being. Therefore, when the provider examines you with their hands, the treatment has already begun. The provider will use different techniques to improve motion after some discussion about the options for treatment and your comfort with the proposed therapy. Among a diverse group of methods, the three most commonly used techniques include

- myofascial release
- isometric stretches, or muscle energy
- high velocity low amplitude treatment

In the use of direct myofascial release, the tissue is loaded with a constant force until release occurs. In indirect myofascial release, the dysfunctional tissues are guided along a path of least resistance until free movement is achieved. It is through the continual direct or indirect engagement of myofascial barriers which the provider palpates that a release of myofascial tissues occurs. For example, myofascial release may relax the myofascial tissue of the low back and a person with chronic pain might improve range of motion.

During isometric stretches, or muscle energy, the person's muscles are actively used against a comparable counterforce by the provider for stretch which might improve the range of motion. The purpose is to restore motion, decrease muscle/tissue changes, and modify asymmetry of somatic dysfunction.

Through high velocity low amplitude treatment, or the thrust technique, the provider employs a rapid and therapeutic force. This force is of short duration and short distance to restore or improve the anatomic range of motion of a joint. The procedure reduces or completely reverses the physical signs of somatic dysfunction tissue changes, asymmetry, restriction of motion, and tenderness. Sometimes during this treatment, you might feel or hear a pop, but success of the technique is not dependent on this experience. Patients will typically have one or two different achievements with spinal manipulation. The first is that they may find instantaneous relief of pain symptoms with the use of spinal manipulation over time. The other is that through motions of spinal manipulation, you will gain confidence that motion can be safe and effective for the body. Before the conclusion of a visit, you and the provider will determine which spinal manipulation techniques worked best for you. You will also decide how many follow-up visits you might need to achieve a desired level of functional improvement. Each person is treated with this shared decision-making perspective in mind.

Energy Medicine

The term "energy medicine" has been in general use since the 1980s. Energy medicine often proposes that imbalances in the body's energy field result in illness. Health can then be restored by rebalancing the body's energy field. Some modalities describe treatments as ridding the body of negative energies or blockages in the mind. Others describe treatment as a release or letting go of a contraction in the mind-body. Energy medicine includes biofield energy healing therapies available in Traditional Chinese Medicine, such as acupuncture, and healing touch.

Traditional Chinese Medicine (TCM)

Traditional Chinese Medicine (TCM) is one of the oldest systems of medicine in history. It is over 3,500 years older than traditional Western medicine like the American Medical Association. TCM is a standardized version of the type of Chinese medicine that was practiced before the Chinese Revolution. It is based on several ancient beliefs. The first is founded on the Daoist belief that the human body is a miniature version of the universe. Another belief is that "Qi," a vital energy that flows through the body, performs multiple functions in maintaining health. Chronic pain results from blockage or imbalance of Qi, and TCM practitioners correct or balance its flow. Other concepts in TCM include the yin/yang and the Five Elements Theories. Concepts such as these are of interest in understanding the history of TCM.

TCM addresses a wide variety of health needs besides pain, including immune enhancement/disease prevention, chemical dependency, anxiety, depression, migraines, maintaining health and wellness, and rehabilitation. TCM practitioners utilize five basic methods of diagnosis in their assessments, including

- inspection (looking)
- auscultation (listening)
- olfaction (smelling)

- inquiry (asking)
- palpation (touching)

A Closer Look

What are the yin/yang and five element theories?

Most people are familiar with the yin/yang symbol. The yin/yang is the harmony between opposing, complementary forces that support health.

In the yin/yang theory, detailed attributions are made regarding the yin or yang character of health. Yin is associated with the parasympathetic nervous system. Yang is associated with the sympathetic nervous system. Examples of opposing forces include

- interior/exterior
- cold/hot
- deficient/excess

- slow/fast
- humidity/dryness
- calm/expressive

The yin/yang illustrates polarity and the notion that one cannot exist without the other.

The five elements symbolically represent the stages of human life and explain the functioning of the body. The theory asserts substances can be divided into one of five basic elements:

- wood
- fire
- water

- metal
- earth

Each contains their own specific characteristics and properties. This theory can be used to describe the movement and the relationship between different elements and phenomena in nature.

Inspection not only focuses on the physical appearance and behavior but also pays particular attention to the tongue. A TCM practitioner's analysis of the tongue will include its size, shape, tension, color, and coating. Often, people are instructed not to brush their tongue prior to an appointment in order to not render the findings obscure. (Yes, you should be cleaning your tongue when you brush your teeth!)

A Closer Look

What are they looking for when they inspect my tongue?

Features of the tongue have several indications:

- Body color indicates the state of blood, organs, and Qi.
- Body shape reflects the state of blood and Qi, and indicates excess or deficiency.
- Body features include texture, spotting, movement, teeth marks, and so on.
- Body moisture reveals the state of fluids in the body.
- Coating indicates the state of organs, especially the stomach.
- Coat thickness includes think, thin, and peeled.
- Body cracks includes the direction of the cracks.
- Coat root indicates impairment of organs if not attached to the tongue's surface.

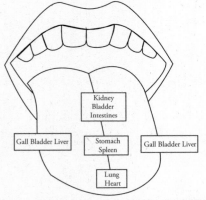

Auscultation refers to listening for particular sounds you make, such as your voice, respiration, and cough.

Olfaction refers to attending to body odor or breath.

During an inquiry, the practitioner will ask ten questions about the regularity, severity, or other characteristics of

- hot/cold symptoms
- perspiration
- the head/face
- pain/tension
- urine/stool
- thirst/appetite
- sleep
- the chest/the abdomen
- gynecological symptoms (if applicable)

The final step in their assessment includes palpation of the wrist pulses at three different locations on the radial artery. The provider will also assess the affected meridians. Meridians are 12 energy pathways that help coordinate the work of the organs and keep the body balanced by regulating its functions.

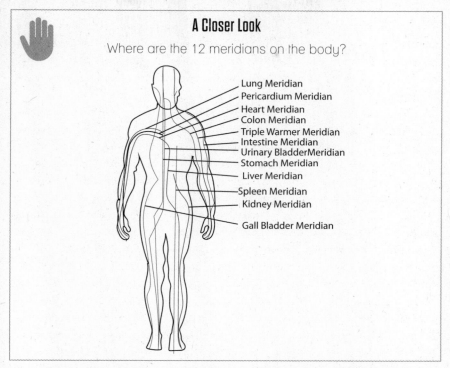

A Closer Look

Where are the 12 meridians on the body?

Lung Meridian
Pericardium Meridian
Heart Meridian
Colon Meridian
Triple Warmer Meridian
Intestine Meridian
Urinary BladderMeridian
Stomach Meridian
Liver Meridian
Spleen Meridian
Kidney Meridian
Gall Bladder Meridian

TCM encompasses several methods designed to help people achieve and maintain health. There are six modern therapeutic methods used in TCM, including moxibustion, tui na massage, cupping/scraping, Chinese herbs, TCM nutrition, and acupuncture.

Moxibustion: A therapy that involves burning moxa, or mugwort root, made from dried artimesia vulgaris (a spongy herb) to facilitate healing. Burning moxa produces a great deal of smoke and a pungent odor, it is often confused with cannabis. The purpose of moxibustion is to

- warm and invigorate the blood
- stimulate the flow of Qi
- strengthen the kidney yang
- expel wind and disperse cold
- dissolve stagnation

There are two types of moxibustion, direct and indirect. In direct moxibustion, a small, cone-shaped amount of moxa is placed on top of an acupuncture needle and burned. You will experience a pleasant heating sensation that penetrates deep into the skin using this technique. Indirect moxibustion is the more popular form of care. In indirect moxibustion, a practitioner lights one end of a moxa stick and holds it close to the area being treated for several minutes until the area turns red. Historically, this therapy had been used to treat menstrual pain. A substitute for moxibustion may be the Teding Diancibo Pu (TDP) lamp, another method of using warming therapy. The TDP lamp has become a new fixture in many practices because it is as effective as moxa. It does not, however, cause respiratory difficulties to sensitive patients. Unlike a traditional heating lamp, the TDP lamp features a plate coated with a mineral formation consisting of 33 elements.

Tui Na Massage: The name comes from two of the actions of the therapy, *tui* meaning "to push" and *na* meaning "to lift and squeeze." Tui na is a combination of massage, acupressure, and other forms of body manipulation. It is a form of Asian bodywork therapy that has been used in China for centuries. In a typical tui na session, you remain clothed and sit on a chair. The practitioner will ask a series of questions and then begin treatment. The type of massage delivered by a tui na practitioner can be quite vigorous at times. Practitioners may sometimes use herbal compresses, ointments, and heat to enhance these techniques. Tui na is best suited for remedying chronic pain and musculoskeletal conditions.

Cupping: During the 2016 Olympic Games in Rio, Michael Phelps made international news when he came out of the pool with circular welts all over his body. It appeared like he had been attacked by an octopus, but instead he had previously had a cupping treatment. Cupping is one of the oldest external methods of TCM. Cupping is a type of Chinese massage, consisting of placing several glass or plastic cups or open spheres on the body. The cups are warmed using a cotton ball or other flammable substance and then placed inside to remove all the oxygen. The substance is then removed before placing the cup against the skin. The air in the cup then cools, creating lower pressure inside the cup. This creates a vacuum and allows the cup to stick to the skin. Fleshy sites on the body are the preferred sites for treatment. Depending on the condition being treated, the cups will be left in place from five to ten minutes. When combined with massage oil, the cups can be slid around the back while drawing up the skin. Drawing up the skin is believed to

- stimulate the flow of blood
- create balance
- realign the flow of Qi
- break up obstructions
- create an avenue for toxins to be drawn out of the body

Gua Sha: Gua Sha, or scraping, is a folk medicine technique that uses pieces of smooth jade, bone, animal tusks, horns, or smooth stones to scrape along the skin to release obstruction and toxins that are trapped at the surface of the skin.

In the United States, some of those materials are not allowed, so they use plastic or glass pieces instead. The scraping is done until red spots begin bruising and cover the treatment area to which it is applied. It is believed that this treatment is for almost any ailment. The red spots and bruising take three to ten days to heal. Often it can be misunderstood by others as a sign of abuse if not informed.

Another alternative is to release blood from the corresponding point of a diseased part of the body using a plum blossom hammer. The hammer has two sides, a dispersed group of needles and a dense group of needles that are hit into the affected area of the body to release the trapped blood.

Chinese Herbology: Practitioners of TCM may also consider using internal medical therapies, such as herbs. The term Chinese herbology can be misleading depending on what substances are being considered. The most commonly used substances can come from different parts of plants. Ginseng is the most broadly used substance for the broadest set of treatments. There are over 13,000 different Chinese medicinals available around the world. *The Chinese Materia Medica* is a pharmacological reference book used by TCM practitioners and describes thousands of medicinal substances. The herbs are combined into a formula that is then distributed in the form of a traditional tea, capsule, liquid extract, granule, or powder. Chinese herbology came to widespread attention in the United States in the 1970s. However, the success of Chinese herbology still remains poorly documented.

Some healthcare professionals hold concerns over a number of potentially toxic Chinese herbs. There are some products that might feel outlandish in the Western hemisphere, but still are considered staple ingredients, such as

- animal products (tiger bones, rhino horns, deer antlers, and snake bile)
- human products (feces, bone, and menstrual blood)
- mineral products (arsenic, asbestos, lead, and mercury)

There have been reports of Chinese herbs being contaminated with drugs, toxins, or heavy metals or not containing the listed ingredients. Some of the herbs used in Chinese medicine can interact with drugs, have serious side effects, or be unsafe for people with certain medical conditions. You should never attempt to take Chinese herbs without proper training or guidance from a licensed practitioner. You should also notify your primary care provider or pharmacist if you are taking Chinese herbs to check for any potential interactions you're your prescription medications.

Chinese Nutrition: Chinese nutrition traditionally was thought of as a lifestyle. It is now considered a mode of dieting rooted in Chinese understandings of the effects of food on the human organism. It was the predominant dietary therapy used before the sciences of biology and chemistry allowed the discovery of present physiological knowledge. It became a therapy for Westerners because of their poor diet. Chinese nutrition is now qualified as integrative health and was introduced and made popular in the Western hemisphere with the release of the book, *The Tao of Healthy Eating*. In Chinese nutrition, a balanced diet is one which includes all five tastes, including

1. spicy (warming)
2. sour (cooling)
3. bitter (cooling)
4. sweet (strengthening)
5. salty (cooling)

Foods that have a particular taste tend to have particular properties. Food items can be classified as heating or cooling, again revisiting the yin/yang concept of TCM. The ratio of these tastes is going to vary according to the individual's needs and the season of the year. Heating foods include red meat, deep-fried goods, and alcohol. It is recommended that heating foods be avoided in the summer and are typically used to treat cold illnesses. Cooling foods include mostly green vegetables. It is recommended that cooling foods be used for hot conditions, such as inflammation. There are no forbidden foods or "one size fits all" diets in TCM. In TCM, nutrition is considered the first line of defense in health matters. At present, it is difficult to determine whether classic TCM diets could influence diseases without any evidence-based research. At the very least, a provider should suggest to their patients to choose more uncontaminated produce and select the least-processed foods when possible.

Acupuncture

Acupuncture is one of the oldest and most commonly used complementary and integrative health treatments in the world. It is part of TCM and is not typically considered a standalone treatment. Despite having originated in China during the Shang Dynasty in 1600–1100 B.C., it has only recently become popular in the Western hemisphere since 1971. Acupuncture began with the discovery that stimulating specific areas of the skin affected the physiological functioning of the body. It has evolved into a scientific system of healing that restores and maintains health. In 1993, the FDA estimated that Americans made 12 million visits per year to acupuncture practitioners. Acupuncture is the practice of inserting and manipulating needles into the superficial skin, subcutaneous tissue, and muscles of the body at particular acupuncture points. In TCM, there are as many as 2,000 acupuncture points on the human body which are connected by the 12 meridians reviewed earlier. These meridians conduct the Qi energy between the surface of the body and its internal organs. Acupuncture is believed to keep the balance between the yin/yang, allowing for the normal flow of Qi associated with neural transmission throughout the body. It also restores health to the mind and body. There is promising scientific evidence to support the use of acupuncture for chronic pain conditions, such as arthritis and headaches, and limited support for neck pain. Acupuncture also tends to provide a short-term effect when compared with a waiting list control or when acupuncture is added to another treatment of chronic low back pain.

Acupuncture is generally safe when administered using clean needles, and practiced by a licensed, trained acupuncturist. Many people express concerns about acupuncture due to their needle phobia. Unlike other needles, acupuncture needles are solid and hair-thin. They are generally inserted no more than a half-inch to an inch depending on the type of treatment being delivered. While each person experiences acupuncture differently, most people feel only a minimal amount of pain as the needles are first inserted. It may take several visits to see significant improvement of the chronic pain condition. Depending on the seriousness and the length of the condition being treated, the traditional acupuncture visit may take between 30 and 60 minutes.

At times, electro-acupuncture may be used to further stimulate the acupuncture points and can be used to replace manipulation of needles. Electroacupuncture is when an electrical current is applied to the needles once they are inserted. It has been found to be especially successful in treating neuromuscular disorders.

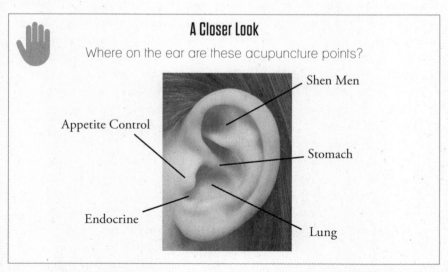

A Closer Look
Where on the ear are these acupuncture points?

Shen Men

Appetite Control

Stomach

Endocrine

Lung

Acupressure and auricular acupuncture may serve as alternatives to people with needle phobia. Acupressure is the application of pressure to key points with the fingers, Auricular acupuncture is the application of small needles, vicaria seeds, pellets, or ear tacks to specific points of the ear. In TCM, the ear is believed to be a microcosm of the body. Each point is related to an anatomical structure and named for their function. The most commonly used points are

- the hunger point for appetite control and weight loss
- the Shen Men, or calming point, for stress management
- the lung point for smoking cessation

Healing Touch

Healing touch is a bio-field therapy that arose in the nursing field in the late 1980s. It is being used in a variety of settings including pain centers with reported benefits. It is an energy-based therapeutic approach to healing that can be used in conjunction with more traditional therapies or as a standalone treatment. It is a contemporary interpretation of several ancient laying-on-of-hands healing practices. The practitioner utilizes non-invasive techniques with their hands to clear, energize, and balance the human and environmental energy fields. This is done in order to facilitate healing at the physical, emotional, mental, and/or spiritual levels. It is based on a heart-centered caring relationship in which you and the practitioner come together energetically to facilitate your health and healing. The goal is to restore balance and harmony in the energy system placing you in a position to self-heal.

Healing touch is based on the assumption that all human beings have the natural ability to heal and enhance healing in others. It is believed that human beings are an open energy system composed of layers of energy that are in constant interaction with self, others, and the environment. Therefore, illness is considered an imbalance in your energy fields, or auras. Energy therapies focus on removing energy congestion that form in the energy tracts and energy centers, or chakras. Once these imbalances and disturbances are cleared, the energy channels resume their task of connecting the body, mind, and spirit to restore health and promote healing.

Most people will inquire about how the healing touch treatment will unfold. The first session usually involves a consultation with a practitioner in addition to an energy session. You will be asked to remain in your hospital bed, sit in a chair, or lay down fully clothed on a massage table in a clinic setting while the practitioner centers themselves mentally. With your permission, the practitioner will then gently place their hands slightly above or on you and begin assessing your energy fields. The practitioner will use their hands to clear and mobilize your energy, direct energy to achieve wholeness, and balance the field. Practitioners may use a number of techniques, including:

- Making a chakra connection (to stimulate movement of energy through the body)
- Mind clearing (to stimulate mental relaxation)
- Magnetic clearing (to cleanse and clear the complete field by removing congested energy and emotional debris)
- Magnetic passes (to provide own personal magnetic fluids through the irradiation of personal energy)

The healing touch session may be implemented at the inpatient bedside in 10 minutes or may be provided in an outpatient clinic over 30 minutes for follow-up or 60 to 90 minutes for intake sessions. People frequently report feeling deeply relaxed and peaceful during and after the session. The practitioner will then evaluate you, ask for feedback, and close the session. There is a cumulative effect of using healing touch over time and regular sessions are recommended. Practitioners say that healing touch is a life-changing gift that can be experienced over and over again.

Healing touch can influence a person's response to pain in many ways. It is interpreted by the body by the physical, emotional, mental, and spiritual aspects of the self. More studies are needed even though research supports the use of healing touch in improving quality of life in chronic disease. The overall outcomes indicate encouraging results for the use of healing touch for pain management specifically. Healing touch has been found to decrease pain in acute, chronic, post-surgical, and centralized sensitization pain conditions. There are no contraindications for using energy work to relieve pain. It can be valuable in supplementing traditional approaches or using when other approaches are not successful. There are several benefits to using healing touch. It is non-invasive, effective, nontoxic, and economical, and it

- restores balance and harmony without medicines
- facilitates the relaxation response
- enhances the healing process
- reduces the need for pain medicine
- helps prevent illness
- enhances a person's spiritual development
- aids in preparation for medical treatments and procedures
- increases energy/relief for chronic fatigue
- supports the dying process

Healing touch does not require the use of equipment or substances and can be done in any setting. An open heart, a set of hands, and a willing spirit are all that are needed.

A Closer Look

Where are the auric bodies and chakras?

Auras have seven layers of elements, including the etheric, the emotional, the mental, the astral, the etheric template, the celestial, and the causal. The energy tracts create a system of energy channels within individuals through which all energy moves throughout the body. There are seven main chakras, including the crown, the third eye, throat, heart, solar plexus, sacral, and base. Chakras are linked together and govern the endocrine system that in turn regulates the aging process. The National Center for Complementary and Integrative Health (NCCIH) notes that the existence of such energy fields has not yet been definitively proven, although scientists are studying these phenomena.

An Introduction to the Aura

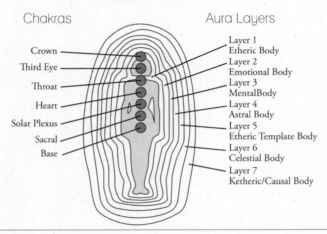

Chakras

Crown
Third Eye
Throat
Heart
Solar Plexus
Sacral
Base

Aura Layers

Layer 1
Etheric Body
Layer 2
Emotional Body
Layer 3
MentalBody
Layer 4
Astral Body
Layer 5
Etheric Template Body
Layer 6
Celestial Body
Layer 7
Ketheric/Causal Body

A Closer Look

Are there any other types of CIH modalities?

There are a number of other CIH modalities available in the market that I did not review in detail here, including:

- Alexander technique: a movement therapy that uses guidance and education on ways to improve posture and movement. The intent is to teach a person how to use muscles more efficiently to improve the overall functioning of the body.
- Ayurveda: A system of medicine that originated in India several thousand years ago. A chief aim of Ayurvedic practices is to cleanse the body of substances that can cause disease, in the belief that this helps to re-establish harmony and balance.

- Chelation therapy: A chemical process in which a substance is used to bind molecules, such as metals or minerals, and hold them tightly so that they can be removed from the body.
- Feldenkrais: A movement therapy that uses a method of education in physical coordination and movement. The intent is to help the person become more aware of how the body moves through space and to improve physical functioning.
- Homeopathy: A system of medical practices based on the theory that any substance that can produce symptoms of disease or illness in a healthy person can cure those symptoms in a sick person.
- Low-level laser therapy (LLLT): A system that utilizes low-power lasers claimed to stimulate tissue and encourage cells to function. There is evidence to support its success in relieving pain conditions, such as rheumatoid arthritis, osteoarthritis, neck pain, and chronic joint disorders.
- Naturopathy: An alternative medical system that proposes that a healing power in the body establishes, maintains, and restores health.
- Pilates: A movement therapy that uses a method of physical exercise to strengthen and build control of muscles, especially those used for posture.
- Reiki: Practitioners use a technique called palm healing or hands-on healing through which a universal energy is transferred through the palms of the practitioner to the patient in order to encourage emotional or physical healing.
- Therapeutic ultrasound: A deep heating modality that is produced by sound waves and then absorbed by body tissues and changed to thermal energy. The effectiveness of therapeutic ultrasound for pain remains questionable.
- Trager: A movement therapy in which practitioners apply a series of gentle, rhythmic rocking movements to the joints. The intent is to release physical tension and increase the body's range of motion.

However, the research on these practices may not be readily available or empirically supported at this time. When patients approach me about using any of the following practices, I share my three common concerns:

1. Are you or anyone you know finding any relief from using this modality?
2. How invasive is this modality? What are the potential side effects?
3. Will getting this treatment break the bank? What are the associated costs?

A Patient Story

A 62-year-old female goes to the pain clinic for about a year and tries all the different modalities available without any relief. The patient has a history of multiple traumas and has suffered two strokes. The current provider introduces her to a nurse who is similar characteristically to her and who has been trained in healing touch. The patient returns a month later and notes that the healing touch is the only thing that has worked for her and that she enjoys working with the nurse.

 Was it the healing touch alone that accounts for the outcome or are there other factors to consider in this outcome? The answers are discussed in chapter 7.

Summary of the Research

There is promising scientific evidence to support the use of CIH for non-cancer pain conditions. Here are some examples (not all covered in this chapter):

- low back pain (cognitive-behavioral therapy, exercise, interdisciplinary rehabilitation, massage, spinal manipulation, yoga, acupuncture, and functional restoration)
- osteoarthritis (acupuncture, tai chi, self-management programs, and walking aids)
- rheumatoid arthritis (omega-3 fatty acids, relaxation, mindfulness meditation, tai chi, and yoga)
- headaches (relaxation training, biofeedback, acupuncture, and spinal manipulation; dietary supplements are promising)
- preliminary for fibromyalgia (tai chi, qi gong, yoga, massage therapy, acupuncture, and balneotherapy)
- promising for irritable bowel syndrome (hypnotherapy and probiotics)
- limited support for neck pain (acupuncture and spinal manipulation)

Conclusion

In chapter 5, I reviewed the complementary and integrative health (CIH) modalities, including exercise and movement therapies, herbs and aromatherapy, spinal manipulation, traditional Chinese medicine, acupuncture, and healing touch. In chapter 6, I discuss the relationship between lifestyle imbalances and chronic pain and review treatments available to address nutrition, functional medicine, weight loss, sleep hygiene, sexual health, vocational rehabilitation, spirituality and religion, traditional healers, and recreation.

References

Abbate S. (2003). Bleeding techniques: Ancient treatments for acupuncture physicians. *Acupuncture Today*, 4, 1–5.

Academy of Traditional Chinese Medicine. (1982). Lectures on essentials of traditional Chinese medicine VI: Methods of diagnosis. *Journal of Traditional Chinese Medicine*, 2, 321–328.

Acupuncture Today. The ABC's of Traditional Chinese Medicine and Acupuncture. Available at: http://www.acupuncturetoday.com/abc/. Accessed on 4/13/15.

Allison N (ed). (1999). *The illustrated encyclopedia of body-mind disciplines.* Rosen Publishing Group.

Altwebmed.com. (2013). Aromatherapy and Pain Management. Available at: altmedweb.com/types/aromatherapy/aromatherapy-and-pain-management. Accessed November 17, 2017.

American Academy of Osteopathy. (1992). An overview of osteopathic manipulation techniques. Available at: http://www.osteohome.com/resources/Articles/Overview_of_OMT.pdf . Accessed November 4, 2009.

Anderson J, Taylor A. Effects of healing touch in clinical practice: A systematic review of randomized clinical trials. *J Holist Nurs*, 2011; 29(3): 221–228.

Arai, Y.C., Ushida, T., Osuga, T., Matsubara, T., Oshima, K., Kawaguchi, K., Kuwabara, C., Nakao, S., Hara, A., Furuta, C., Aida, E., Ra, S., Takagi, Y., Watakabe, K. (2008). The effect of acupressure at the extra 1 point on subjective and autonomic responses to needle insertion. *Anesth Analg.* 107(2), 661–4.

Barnes, P.M., Bloom, B., Nahin, R. (2008). Complementary and Alternative Medicine Use Among Adults and Children: United States, 2007, CDC National Health Statistics Report #12. Retrieved April 7, 2009, from Centers for Disease Control Web site: http://www.cdc.gov/nchs/data/nhsr/nhsr012.pdf

Beal M (ed). (2009). The principles of palpatory diagnosis and manipulative technique. American Academy of Osteopathy Affiliated with the American Osteopathic Association. Available at: http://www.iahe.com/images/pdf/Description_of_fifty_diagnostic_tests_used_with_osteopathic_manipulation.pdf. Accessed August 12, 2015.

Bell, J. (2008). Massage therapy helps to increase range of motion, decrease pain and assist in healing a client with low back pain and sciatica symptoms. *J Bodyw Mov Ther.* 12(3), 281–9.

Boundless. (2015). The first law: Inertia. Boundless physics. Available at: https://www.boundless.com/physics/textbooks/boundless-physics-textbook/the-laws-of-motion-4/newton-s-laws-46/the-first-law-inertia-236-10947/. Accessed August 12, 2015.

Brady, L.H., Henry, K., Luth, J.F. 2nd, Casper-Bruett, K.K. (2001). The effects of shiatsu on lower back pain. *J Holist Nurs.* 19(1), 57–70.

Brown C, Barner J, Richards K, et al. Patterns of complementary and alternative medicine use in African Americans. *J Altern Complement Med*, 2007; 13(7): 751–758.

Chen, H.M., Chang, F.Y., Hsu, C.T. (2005). Effect of acupressure on nausea, vomiting, anxiety and pain among post-cesarean section women in Taiwan. *Kaohsiung J Med Sci.* 21(8), 341–50.

Cheng X. (1987). *Chinese acupuncture and moxibustion (1st ed).* Foreign Languages Press.

Cherkin, D.C., Eisenberg, D., Sherman, K.J., Barlow, W., Kaptchuk, T.J., Street, J., Deyo, R.A. (2001). Randomized trial comparing traditional Chinese medical acupuncture, therapeutic massage, and self-care education for chronic low back pain. *Arch Intern Med.* 161(8), 1081–8.

Chinese Medicine Living. What is Traditional Chinese Medicine? Available at: http://www.chinesemedicineliving.com/blog/medicine/traditional-chinese-medicine. Accessed on 4/13/15.

Cordes P, Proffitt C, Roth J. The effect of healing touch therapy on the pain and joint mobility experienced by patients with total knee replacements. 2002. In *Healing Touch Research Survey.* Lakewood, CO: Healing Touch International.

Craig K. *Biopsychosocial approach in pain management: A case study.* 2012. Available at: http://www.nilpain.org/ webstorage/webstorage5/ Biopsychosocial%20approach%20in%20pain%20management%20-%20 a%20case %20study %20hypothesis ..pdf. Accessed March 12, 2013.

Creating Healing Relationships. *Healing Touch Program.* 2012. Available at: http://www. Healingtouch program.com/ about/what-is-healing-touch. Accessed October 5, 2012.

Currin, J., Meister, E.A. (2008). A hospital-based intervention using massage to reduce distress among oncology patients. *Cancer Nurs.* 31(3), 214–21.

Daenen L, Varkey E, Kellmann M, et al. (2014). Exercise, not to exercise, or how to exercise in patients with chronic pain? Applying science to practice. *Clinical Journal of Pain.* Available at: http://www.researchgate.net/profile/Liesbeth_Daenen/publication/261067756_Exercise_not_to_Exercise_or_how_to_Exercise_in_Patients_with_Chronic_Pain_Applying_Science_to_Practice/links/5412136e0cf2fa878ad3967c.pdf. Accessed May 18, 2015.

Darbonne M. *The effect of HT modalities on patients with chronic pain.* 1997. Natchitoches, LA: Northwestern State University.

Destefano L. (2011). *Greenman's principles of manual medicine.* Lippincott Williams & Wilkins.

Diener D. A pilot study of the effect of chakra connection and magnetic unruffle on perception of pain in people with fibromyalgia. Healing Touch Newsletter, Research Edition, 2001; 01(3): 7–8.

Dryden, T., Baskwill, A., Preyde, M. (2004). Massage therapy for the orthopaedic patient: a review. *Orthop Nurs.* 23(5), 327–32.

Engelhardt U. (2001). Dietetics in Tang China and the first extant works of material dietetica. In Hsu E (ed.), *Innovation in Chinese Medicine*, Cambridge: Cambridge University Press.

Field, T., Figueiredo, B., Hernandez-Reif, M., Diego, M., Deeds, O., Ascencio, A. (2008). Massage therapy reduces pain in pregnant women, alleviates prenatal depression in both parents and improves their relationships., *J Bodyw Mov Ther.* 12(2), 146–50.

Flaws B. (1999). *The Tao of healthy eating: Dietary wisdom according to traditional Chinese medicine (2nd ed).* Blue Poppy Press.

Franke H, Franke J, Fryer G. (2014). Osteopathic manipulative treatment for nonspecific low back pain: A systematic review and meta-analysis. *BMC Musculoskeletal Disorders, 15,* 286.

Frey Law, L.A., Evans, S., Knudtson, J. Nus, S., Scholl, K., Sluka, K.A. (2008). Massage reduces pain perception and hyperalgesia in experimental muscle pain: a randomized, controlled trial. *J Pain.* 9(8), 714–21.

Gugliemo W. (1998). Are D.O.s losing their unique identity? *Medical Economics, 75,* 201–213.

Hattan, J., King, L., Griffiths, P. (2002). The impact of foot massage and guided relaxation following cardiac surgery: a randomized controlled trial. *J Adv Nurs.* 37(2), 199–207.

Hsieh, L.L., Kuo, C.H., Lee, L.H., Yen, A.M., Chien, K.L., Chen, T.H. (2006). Treatment of low back pain by acupressure and physical therapy: randomised controlled trial. *BMJ.* 332(7543), 696–700.

Hughes, D., Ladas, E., Rooney, D., Kelly, K. (2008). Massage therapy as a supportive care intervention for children with cancer, *Oncol Nurs Forum.* 35(3), 431–42.

Hulme, J., Waterman, H., Hillier, V.F. (1999). The effect of foot massage on patients' perception of care following laparoscopic sterilization as day case patients. *J Adv Nurs.* 30(2), 460–8.

Institute for Traditional Medicine. Cupping. Available at: http://www.itmonline.org/arts/cupping.htm. Accessed on 3/28/14.

Jane, S.W., Wilkie, D.J., Gallucci, B.B., Beaton, R.D., Huang, S.H.Y., (2008). Effects of a Full-Body Massage on Pain Intensity, Anxiety, and Physiological Relaxation in Taiwanese Patients with Metastatic Bone Pain: A Pilot Study. *J Pain Symptom Manage.* 37(4):754–63.

Johnson S, Kurtz M, Kurtz J. (1997). Variables influencing the use of osteopathic manipulative treatment in family practice. *Journal of the American Osteopathic Association, 97,* 80–87.

Konlian C. (1998). Aquatic therapy: Making a wave in the treatment of low back injuries. Orthopaedic Nursing: PDF only. Available at: http://journals.lww.com/orthopaedicnursing/Abstract/1999/01000/Aquatic_Therapy__Making_a_Wave_in_the_Treatment_of.4.aspx.

Kshettry, V.R., Carole, L.F., Henly, S.J., Sendelbach, S., Kummer, B. (2006). Complementary alternative medical therapies for heart surgery patients: feasibility, safety, and impact. *Ann Thorac Surg.* 81(1), 201

Lang, T., Hager, H., Funovits, V., Barker, R., Steinlechner, B., Hoerauf, K., Kober, A. (2007). Prehospital analgesia with acupressure at the Baihui and Hegu points in patients with radial fractures: a prospective, randomized, double-blind trial. *Am J Emerg Med.* 25(8), 887–93.

Le Blanc-Louvry, I., Costaglioli, B., Boulon, C., Leroi, A.M., Ducrotte, P. (2002). Does mechanical massage of the abdominal wall after colectomy reduce postoperative pain and shorten the duration of ileus? Results of a randomized study. *J Gastrointest Surg.* 6(1), 43–9.

Lee M, Ernst E. (2011). Acupuncture for pain: An overview of Cochrane reviews. *Chinese Journal of Integrative Medicine, 17,* 187–189.

Lytle C. (1993). *An Overview of Acupuncture.* Washington, DC: United States Department of Health and Human Services, Health Sciences Branch, Division of Life Sciences, Office of Science and Technology, Center for Devices and Radiological Health, Food and Drug Administration.

Mehling, W.E., Jacobs, B., Acree, M., Wilson, L., Bostrom, A., West, J., Acquah, J., Burns, B., Chapman, J., Hecht, F.M. (2007). Symptom management with massage and acupuncture in postoperative cancer patients: a randomized controlled trial. *J Pain Symptom Manage.* 33(3), 258–66.

Mohammed, G. (2002). Catnip and Kerosene Grass: What Plants Teach Us About Life. Candlenut Books.

Moraska, A., Chandler, C. (2008). Changes in Clinical Parameters in Patients with Tension-type Headache Following Massage Therapy: A Pilot Study. *J Man Manip Ther.* 16(2), 106–12.

Moraska, A., Chandler, C., Edmiston-Schaetzel, A., Franklin, G., Calenda, E.L., Enebo, B. (2008). Comparison of a targeted and general massage protocol on strength, function, and symptoms associated with carpal tunnel syndrome: a randomized pilot study. *J Altern Complement Med.* 14(3), 259–67.

Mornhinweg G, Voignier R. (1995). Holistic Nursing Interventions. Orthopedic Nursing, PDF only. Available at: http://journals.lww.com/orthopaedicnursing/Abstract/1995/07000/Holistic_Nursing_Interventions.4.aspx.

Nahin, R., Barnes, P., Stussman, B. & Bloom, B. (2009). Costs of Complementary and Alternative Medicine and Frequency of Visits to CAM Practitioners: US, 2007. US Department of Health & Human Services. National Health Statistics Report.

National Center for Complementary & Alternative Medicine (NCCAM). Chronic pain and complementary health practices. Available at: http://nccam.nih.gov/health/providers/digest/chronicpain.htm. Accessed February 5, 2014.

National Center for Complementary and Integrative Health. Traditional Chinese Medicine: An Introduction. Available at: https://nccih.nih.gov/health/whatiscam/chinesemed.htm. Accessed on 10/21/11.

Natural Health Way. How TDP infrared lamps work to speed healing. Available at: http://naturalhealthway.com/tdplamps/how-tdp-lamps-work.html. Accessed on 4/13/15.

Nielsen A. (1995). *Gua Sha: A traditional technique for modern practice*. Churchill Livingstone.

Nixon, M., Teschendorff, J., Finney, J., Karnilowicz, W. (1997). Expanding the nursing repertoire: the effect of massage on post-operative pain. *Aust J Adv Nurs*. 14(3), 21–6.

Osteopathic Healthcare of Maine. (2015). Comparison of osteopathic physicians, allopathic physicians, and chiropractors. Available at: http://osteopathichealthcareofmaine.com/osteopathy/do-vs-md-and-dc. Accessed August 12, 2015.

Pettman E. (2007). A history of manipulative therapy. *Journal of Manual & Manipulative Therapy*, 15, 165–174.

Piotrowski, M.M., Paterson, C., Mitchinson, A., Kim, H.M., Kirsh, M., Hinshaw, D.B. (2003). Massage as adjuvant therapy in the management of acute postoperative pain: a preliminary study in men. *J Am Coll Surg*. 197(6), 1037–46.

Quinn, F., Hughes, C.M., Baxter, G.D. (2008). Reflexology in the management of low back pain: a pilot randomised controlled trial. *Complement Ther Med*. 16(1), 3–8.

Robertson V, Robertson V, Low J, et al. (2006). *Electrotherapy explained: Principles and practice*. Elsevier Health Sciences.

Sagar, S.M., Dryden, T., Wong, R.K. (2007). Massage therapy for cancer patients: a reciprocal relationship between body and mind. *Curr Oncol*. 14(2), 45–56

Santrock, J. *A topical approach to human life-span development (3rd edition)*. St. Louis, MO: McGraw-Hill; 2007.

Schatz C. Mindfulness meditation improves connections in the brain. *Harvard Women's Health Watch*, April 08, 2011.

Seers, K., Crichton, N., Martin, J., Coulson, K., Carroll, D. (2008). A randomised controlled trial to assess the effectiveness of a single session of nurse administered massage for short term relief of chronic non-malignant pain. *BMC Nurs*. 7, 10.

Shang A, Huwiler K, Nartey L, et al. (2007). Placebo-controlled trials of Chinese herbal medicine and conventional medicine comparative study. *International Journal of Epidemiology*, 36, 1086–1092.

Slater V. *Safety, elements, and effects of healing touch on chronic non-malignant abdominal pain*. 1996. Unpublished doctoral dissertation, University of Tennessee, College of Nursing, Knoxville, TN.

Still J. (2003). Use of animal products in traditional Chinese medicine: Environmental impact and health hazards. *Complementary Therapies in Medicine, 11*, 118–122.

Suresh, S., Wang, S., Porfyris, S., Kamasinski-Sol, R., Steinhorn, D.M. (2008). Massage therapy in outpatient pediatric chronic pain patients: do they facilitate significant reductions in levels of distress, pain, tension, discomfort, and mood alterations?, *Paediatr Anaesth*. 18(9), 884–7.

Taylor, A.G., Galper, D.I., Taylor, P., Rice, L.W., Andersen, W., Irvin, W., Wang, X.Q., Harrell, F.E. Jr. (2003). Effects of adjunctive Swedish massage and vibration therapy on short-term postoperative outcomes: a randomized, controlled trial. *J Altern Complement Med*. 9(1), 77–89.

The American College of Traditional Chinese Medicine. Clinical Manual. Available at: http://www.actcm.edu/wp-content/uploads/2014/07/Clinic-Manual-2013-2014.pdf. Accessed on 3/28/14.

Veith I, Rose K. (2002). *The yellow emperor's classic of internal medicine*. University of California Press.

Walach, H., Güthlin, C., König, M. (2003). Efficacy of massage therapy in chronic pain: a pragmatic randomized trial. *J Altern Complement Med*. 9(6), 837–46.

Wang, H.L., Keck, J.F. (2004). Foot and hand massage as an intervention for postoperative pain. *Pain Manag Nurs*. 5(2), 59–65.

Wardell D, Weymouth K. Review of studies of healing touch. *J Nurs Scholarsh*, 2004; 36(2): 147–154.

Wardell D. The trauma release technique: How it is taught and experienced in healing touch. *Altern Complement Ther*, 2000; 6(1): 20–27.

Xu S, et al. (2013). Adverse events of acupuncture: A systematic review of case reports. *Evidence Based Complementary and Alternative Medicine*, 1.

Yu B, Gong X. (2011). Necessary conditions for the globalization of traditional Chinese medicine. *Journal of Chinese Integrative Medicine, 9*, 341–348.

Zhu Y. (1998). *Chinese Materia Medica: Chemistry, Pharmacology and Applications (1st ed)*. CRC Press.

Chapter 6

Lifestyle Imbalance Management

Chronic pain tends to negatively affect your level of stress, mood, and substance use as described in chapter 2, but it also affects the following areas of your life:

- nutrition
- weight
- sleep
- sexual health
- vocational rehabilitation
- spirituality
- recreation

This chapter discusses the importance of maintaining a balance in your lifestyle. Traditional approaches are often the first option to fix something fickle before we even look at the potential behind lifestyle changes. Often, this is an area that is ignored or taken for granted. By addressing these areas, you may be also indirectly addressing your pain. These areas have a mutual relationship with your pain.

Questions for the Reader to Ponder

By the end of this chapter, you should be able to answer the following questions:

1. What foods are beneficial to people with joint pain?
2. How are pain and sex related?
3. Why would you access vocational rehabilitation services?
4. Can prescribed medications used to relieve pain fragment sleep?
5. Can your spirituality give you purpose in your life despite being in pain?
6. Which activities does recreation therapy include?

Nutrition

"Mother Nature is the best pharmacist and food is the most powerful drug on the planet." —Mark Hyman

A nutritional approach to pain management involves making changes to your diet. This is done to prevent pain or promote the relief of inflammation as part of a comprehensive pain management strategy. Back/joint pain, rheumatoid arthritis, fibromyalgia, and osteoarthritis are affected by your diet.

Researchers have highlighted the advantages of certain foods when added to one's diet. They have suggested avoiding foods thought to contribute to chronic pain. After one month of avoiding these foods, a consecutive reintroduction of each particular food every couple of days can follow. For example, a person diagnosed with gout may need help decreasing uric acid levels in their blood. Limiting their intake of high purine foods may help to decrease their joint pain. According to the American Medical Association, purine containing foods include beer, anchovies, yeast, organ meat, legumes, meat gravies, mushrooms, spinach, asparagus, and cauliflower. Foods which may decrease inflammation and be beneficial to people with gout include dark berries, tofu, salmon, olive oil, and nuts. Essential fatty acids, like omega-3, regulate inflammatory responses. They are believed to help with rheumatoid arthritis and fibromyalgia. Common sources of omega-3 fatty acids include flax seeds, walnuts, cold-water fish, and soybeans. Foods that may help control chronic pain in conditions such as rheumatoid arthritis and fibromyalgia include cherries, soy, oranges, peaches, asparagus, cranberries, cauliflower, and kiwi. There are foods that theoretically worsen inflammation and consumption and should be decreased, including dairy products, chocolate, eggs, meat, wheat, corn, and nuts. In reference to osteoarthritis, people should make sure to have plenty of vitamin D and calcium in their diet. Food sources of vitamin D include salmon, tuna, mackerel, and milk, orange juice, and yogurt with added vitamin D. There are additional steps people can follow to obtain more vitamin D, such as receiving more mid-day sun exposure and taking supplements.

Food sources of calcium include milk products, beans, tofu, nuts, meats, fish, poultry, oats/grains, orange juice, soy, broccoli, turnip greens, okra, and kale. Nutritional health can also provide relief for constipation caused by opioid pain medications and muscle relaxants. A typical health plan may include

1. Eating a high-fiber diet, which includes foods such as fruits, vegetables, whole grains, seeds, and beans
2. Drinking about eight glasses of water daily
3. Avoiding coffee drinks, whole milk, and sodas as they contribute to constipation
4. Reducing eating foods that cause constipation, including cheese, ice cream, whole milk, fatty meats, sugar processed foods, and pastries
5. Eating foods like papaya and some yogurt products
6. Exercising regularly
7. Reducing stress

8. Assuming a squatting position at the toilet
9. Taking time for healthy elimination
10. Having a prophylactic bowel regimen

A Closer Look

Which diet is right for me?

People who suffer from chronic pain may have stumbled upon any number of "pain-lowering" diets while surfing the internet, such as the

- Atkins diet: A diet emphasizing a drastic reduction in the daily intake of carbohydrates (40 grams or less), countered by an increase in protein and fat.
- Macrobiotic diet: A diet low in fat, emphasizing whole grains and vegetables and restricting the intake of fluids.
- Ornish diet: A high-fiber, low-fat vegetarian diet that promotes weight loss and health by controlling what is eaten, not by restricting the intake of calories.
- Pritikin diet: A low-fat diet that allows meat but emphasizes the consumption of foods with a large volume of fiber and water.
- South Beach diet: A diet that distinguishes between "good" and "bad" carbohydrates and fats. Dieters are encouraged to eat whole-grain foods and an abundant amount of vegetables.
- Vegetarian diet: Diets that are totally devoid of meat, red or white. Numerous variations are followed on the nonmeat theme.
- Zone diet: A diet in which each meal consists of a small amount of low-fat protein, fats, and fiber-rich fruits and vegetables. Its basic goal is to alter the body's metabolism by controlling the production of key hormones.

However, there continues to be no standard guideline for nutritional health to address pain.

A basic principle of nutritional health is to eat food from each of the basic food groups every day. The Food Guide Pyramid was introduced by the US Department of Agriculture in 1992. It was then updated in 2005 to Mypyramid. gov because the original pyramid was too misleading and hard to understand. The Mypyramid.gov movement was eventually replaced by MyPlate in 2011. The plate was advised by the then First Lady's anti-obesity team and federal health officials.

A Closer Look

How are the different food programs different?

The original Food Guide Pyramid was divided into six horizontal sections containing depictions of foods from each section's group.

The six groups were as follows:

1. fats, oils, and sweets (used sparingly)
2. milk, yogurt, and cheese (2–3 servings)
3. meat, poultry, fish, dry beans, eggs, and nuts (2–3 servings)
4. vegetables (3–5 servings)
5. fruits (2–4 servings)
6. bread, cereal, rice, and pasta (6–11 servings)

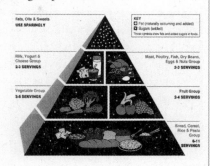

Mypyramid.gov had colorful vertical wedges replacing the horizontal sections and was often displayed without the food images in an abstract design.

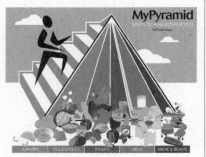

Now there is a plate that is split into four slightly different sized quadrants, with fruits and vegetables taking up half the space, and grains and protein making up the other half. People are recommended to fill at least half the grain space with whole grains. The vegetables and grains portions are the largest of the four. A smaller circle sits beside the plate for dairy products.

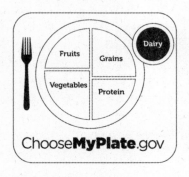

Functional Medicine

Numerous things can contribute to chronic pain, including diet, exercise, thoughts, feelings, and environmental toxins. Science has proven what we may have known intuitively—how we live, the quality of our relationships, the food we eat, and how we use our bodies determines much more than our genes ever will. In other words, we are treating the chronic pain by addressing these poor habits. This is also a fundamental principle of sustainable health. According to the American College of Preventative Medicine, most chronic diseases are preventable and reversible if a comprehensive, individualized approach is implemented. This approach addresses genetics, diet, nutrition, stress, exercise, and sleep through integrated "functional medicine" teams and based on empirical research.

Functional medicine (FM) addresses the underlying causes of disease, using a systems-oriented approach. FM engages both the patient and the practitioner in a therapeutic partnership. The "I" in illness underlines how disease affects the body or mind of the individual. The "W" in wellness directs us to work together to reach a state of being in good physical and mental health. In a word, it is the medicine of "why, not what." FM is further guided by six core principles:

1. An understanding of the biochemical individuality of each person, based on the concepts of genetics and environmental influence
2. Emphasis on a patient-centered rather than a disease-centered approach to treatment
3. A search for a dynamic balance among the internal and external
4. Familiarity with the complex connections of internal physiological factors
5. The identification of health as a positive vitality not merely the absence of disease
6. The promotion of organ preservation as the means to enhance the health span, not just the lifespan, of each individual

The role of FM practitioners is to spend time with their patients, listening to their histories. They look at the interactions among factors that influence long-term health and chronic disease. FM practitioners can help prevent, treat, and often cure chronic conditions more successfully and at lower cost than traditional medicine. One way which FM providers can do this is to guide patients on the implementation of a modified, elimination, anti-inflammatory diet. It is important to remember that every time we eat, we are changing our body chemistry. People are taught to

- remove all added sugars
- remove foods containing gluten or dairy
- consume more vegetables and fruits that cover every color of the rainbow
- consume healthy fats, protein, nuts and seeds, legumes and beverages
- consume meats that are organic, wild caught, and grass-fed

Basically, people are recommended to eat only *real* food and to eat mindfully. Additional specific foods may be removed from the diet to uncover if they are potential causes of adverse food reactions. Some reactions can occur immediately after eating a food such as an allergy. In other cases, the reaction can be delayed by hours to days, such as an intolerance or sensitivity. Use of an elimination, anti-inflammatory diet will ask you to remove some of the most common causes of food sensitivity while monitoring your medical symptoms to see if there is an improvement. You will follow this dietary lifestyle for three weeks and log the changes that occur with your body. It is important that you have bowels and urine flowing. You will need to read and understand food labels, inquire the Internet, or ask your providers about ingredients. At the end of three weeks, you will then be asked if you would like to go back to your former dietary lifestyle or if you would like to continue the detoxification process. If you choose to keep most foods out of your diet, you will be encouraged to add specific foods back into the diet for one to two days with monitoring of symptoms. If you do not experience symptoms of sensitivity, that specific food can stay in your diet if it is a good source of nutrition.

A Closer Look

How do you practice mindful eating?

If you have heard about mindful eating but aren't sure where or how to start, here are instructions for a brief mindfulness eating exercise. The following exercise is simple and will only take a few minutes.

1. Find a small piece of food, such as a baby carrot or a nut.
2. Begin by exploring this little piece of food, using as many of your senses as possible.
3. Look at the food. Notice its texture. Notice its color.
4. Now, close your eyes, and explore the food with your sense of touch. What does this food feel like? Is it hard or soft? Grainy or sticky? Moist or dry?
5. Before you eat, explore this food with your sense of smell. What do you notice?
6. Now, take your first bite. Please chew very slowly, noticing the actual sensory experience of chewing and tasting. You might want to close your eyes for a moment.
7. Notice the texture of the food; the way it feels in your mouth.
8. Notice if the intensity of its flavor changes, moment to moment.
9. Take about 20 more seconds to very slowly finish this first bite of food.
10. Now, please take your second and last bite. As before, chew very slowly, while paying close attention to the actual sensory experience of eating.

Weight Loss

According to the CDC, about two-thirds of US adults are overweight or obese and are at increased risk for musculoskeletal disease. The US has witnessed a shift in averages in reference to weight in the past few decades. The first lineman in an American football team over 300 pounds was William "The Refrigerator" Perry (355 pounds) in 1960. Today, the average weight of every lineman in the national football league is 355 pounds, with a life expectancy of about 57 years. Healthcare claims have estimated the coexistence of pain and obesity to be as high as 30%. These high rates are related to decreased quality of life, emotional distress, increased disability, sedentary lifestyle, and stigma.

Past research suggests that there is a direct relationship between weight and frequency of musculoskeletal pain. Rates of neck, back, hip, knee, and ankle pain have been found to be significantly higher in obese individuals. An underlying relationship remains unclear. Similar to the chicken or the egg dilemma, it is yet unknown whether obesity causes pain or vice versa. Obesity is assumed to lead to knee and low back pain because of excess mechanical stresses. Fat functions much like an organ that secretes chemicals which affect blood pressure and cholesterol. Carrying five pounds of extra weight feels like ten pounds on your body's joints. Ten pounds feels like twenty pounds on your joints, especially the knees. Obesity has been related with thoracic spine, neck, and upper extremity pain. It has also been linked with conditions such as fibromyalgia, migraines, and headaches due to its pro-inflammatory state. Chronic pain may also result in obesity because of physical inactivity and emotional eating. The opposite must be true—weight loss can reduce chronic pain. One study found that more than a 10% loss of body weight from diet alone resulted in a 50% decrease in knee osteoarthritis in obese people. When you reach a 10% weight loss, the levels of inflammatory substances circulating in your blood will drop significantly.

The problem with reducing weight is complicated. Chances are, people who suffer from chronic pain are unable to move or exercise enough to lose weight. Medications, such as opioids, sedatives, muscle relaxants, or antidepressants, may suppress the body's metabolism and contribute to weight gain. These co-occurring diseases both respond to behavioral self-management interventions.

An integrative approach that combines nutrition, physical activity, and behavioral strategies appears to provide maximum benefit. A nutritional intervention may include classes on topics related to

- improving food consumption
- reading nutrition facts labels
- learning portion control
- completing of dietary records

- having individual consultations with a nutritional health provider

When reading nutrition facts, people are taught to discriminate the information listed on the label of the food product. The information in the main or top section contains product-specific information such as serving size, calories, and nutrient information. The bottom section contains a footnote with daily values for 2,000 and 2,500 calorie diets, which provides recommended dietary information for important nutrients including fats, sodium, and fiber. People also learn several tips for controlling portion sizes, including:

1. Avoiding skipping meals and eating at regular intervals
2. Using measuring cups and food weight scales
3. Knowing rules about serving sizes
4. Knowing the difference between serving versus portion size listed on nutrition facts labels
5. Using portion control plates
6. Developing good "eating out" habits
7. Planning your meals
8. Using smaller plates

When using a dietary record approach, you record the foods and beverages and the amounts consumed over one or more days. Ideally, the recording is done at the time of eating in order to avoid reliance on memory. You then return for an individual consultation with a nutritional health provider to review your progress.

A Quick Portion Guide

Food Portion	20 Years Ago	Food Portion	Now
3-inch Bagel 140 calories		6-inch Bagel 350 calories	
Cheeseburger 333 calories		Cheeseburger 590 calories	
French Fries 2.4 ounces 210 calories		French Fries 6.9 ounces 610 calories	

Soda 6.5 ounces 85 calories		Soda 20 ounces 250 calories	
Coffee (with whole milk and sugar) 8 ounces 45 calories		Mocha Coffee (with steamed whole milk and mocha syrup) 16 ounces 350 calories	
Pepperoni Pizza (pictured) 500 calories		Pepperoni Pizza 850 calories	
Chicken Caesar Salad 1.5 cups 390 calories		Chicken Caesar Salad 3.5 cups 790 calories	
Popcorn 5 cups 270 calories		Popcorn 11 cups 630 calories	
Chocolate Chip Cookie 1.5-inch diameter 55 calories		Chocolate Chip Cookie 3.5-inch diameter 275 calories	
Chicken Stir Fry 2 cups 435 calories		Chicken Stir Fry 4.5 cups 865 calories	

Psychological interventions often focus on behavioral and cognitive strategies for weight management. Research shows that behavioral interventions tend to be more successful than cognitive treatments. Strategies might include

- self-monitoring
- controlling stimuli
- goal setting
- problem-solving
- identifying antecedents, behaviors, and consequences

Other than medication and surgery, cognitive-behavioral therapy (CBT) has been shown to be an effective treatment for weight loss. A psychological intervention may include

- the assessment and diagnosis of mental problems most commonly associated with obesity
- the provision of therapy support groups
- short-term individual psychological therapy

Research findings suggest that obesity is resistant to long-term psychological methods of treatment, such as CBT. Not everyone is lucky enough to be able to attend a multidisciplinary weight management program. Primary care providers are often the front-line practitioners of the obesity epidemic. Often, they may overlook this disease due to time constraints, being unfamiliar with treatment options, and focusing on other treatable conditions.

Sleep Hygiene

There are about ten different sleep disorders, including narcolepsy, restless leg syndrome, obstructive sleep apnea, and insomnia. Excessive daytime sleepiness is a symptom that can occur with several sleep disorders. Excessive daytime sleepiness may include episodes of uncontrolled sleep attacks that occur while in conversation, reading, watching television, or driving. Excessive daytime sleepiness may be caused by not getting enough hours of quality sleep. Adults between 26 and 64 years of age need about 7 to 9 hours of sleep per day. Disturbed sleep can have many health consequences, including fatigue, decreased focus, and altered mood, and can be a potential warning sign for osteoarthritis.

About two-thirds of people who suffer from chronic pain also report poor sleep due to the relationship between these two conditions. The problem of pain and sleep becomes even more complicated because many medications commonly prescribed to relieve pain (oxycodone, morphine, and codeine) can fragment sleep. If you experience poor sleep due to pain one night, you will likely experience more pain the next night and so on, creating a vicious cycle. Chronic pain frequently is associated with a sleep disorder and these coexisting problems can be difficult to treat.

Sleep disorders are diagnosed through a comprehensive assessment that includes a detailed patient history, physical exam, questionnaires, sleep diaries, and sleep studies. During a typical sleep study, you will be connected to testing equipment that measure various biological functions, including

- brain activity
- muscle activity
- respiratory effort
- eye movements

- heart rhythm
- oxygen saturation
- sleep latency, duration, and efficiency

The temperature of the room is maintained at comfortable level and the lights are turned off. After the study is completed, you will follow up with a specialist to review the outcomes and develop a treatment plan.

Narcolepsy: A neurologic disorder involving the loss of the brain's ability to regulate sleep cycles normally. People with this condition experience frequent excessive daytime sleepiness and disturbed nighttime sleep. They generally experience the rapid eye movement (REM) stage of sleep within five minutes of falling asleep. They also tend to experience difficulties staying asleep. They may have a sudden and passing episode of muscle weakness accompanied by full conscious awareness. This is typically triggered by emotions. Some people may suffer from the temporary inability to move or speak while falling asleep or waking. This may be accompanied by hallucinations. After developing narcolepsy, many people suddenly gain weight, which can be prevented by active treatment.

Restless Leg Syndrome: A creeping, crawling, tingling, aching, burning, pulling, and cramping in the calves, thighs, feet, or arms. The sensation commonly is relieved by movement of the legs or walking around. When movement stops, the sensations frequently return. The abnormal sensations are more common in the late afternoon or evening hours. This condition can disrupt sleep, leading to daytime drowsiness. It affects about 10% of the US population. Prescription medications are available to reduce the restlessness. Self-care, coping skills, and avoidance of caffeine can help reduce symptoms.

Obstructive Sleep Apnea: An extreme form of snoring in which a person's airway becomes partially or completely blocked several times during the night. This leads to repetitive arousals without any recollection and disrupted sleep. Approximately 2% of women and 4% of men in the US suffer from the condition. There are several potential risk factors, including obesity, inherited traits, and use of alcohol before sleep. If left untreated, this condition can lead to high blood pressure, heart disease, changes in mood, memory problems, and death. There are a variety of treatment options available if underlying health issues or environmental factors cannot be identified or changed. Treatments include

- weight loss
- sleep positioning (do not sleep on the back)
- dental devices
- surgical procedures

The most common and efficacious way of treating this disorder is by using a continuous positive airway pressure (CPAP) device. A CPAP device works by blowing a steady stream of air into the nose through a mask. This prevents pauses in breathing during sleep. CPAP is mostly delivered through a nasal mask, but oral and naso-oral masks often are used when nasal congestion or obstruction is an issue. The success of CPAP depends on user compliance. If the wearer does not put on the device, it will not work. People tend to become noncompliant when the CPAP mask is the wrong size or style, causing skin irritation or pressure sores. The CPAP device needs to fit properly. Some people have trouble adapting to the mask for various reasons:

- the forced air from the CPAP that causes dry mouth or a stuffy nose
- claustrophobia
- difficulty falling asleep with the mask on
- unintentionally removing the mask during the night
- being annoyed by the noise of the device

Another concern related to the use of CPAP is its cleaning and maintenance. People are unaware of the need for daily cleaning of the tubing, mask, and headgear in warm soapy water with a mild dish detergent. People should also wipe down the device with a damp cloth and wash the filter at the back of the machine with tap water weekly. The mask, tubing, and filters will need to be replaced after wear and tear. In addition, there are six steps to help you with the general maintenance of your CPAP device:

1. Make cleaning your device part of your routine, allowing the equipment ample time to dry
2. Keep the machine and accessories out of direct sunlight to avoid damage
3. Never use bleach to clean accessories. Always use distilled or sterile water when cleaning components
4. Replace power cords and data cards due to equipment malfunctions
5. Place the device on a level surface away from objects such as curtains that may interfere with air intake
6. Keep track of when you need to order replacement parts to get the most out of therapy

Insomnia: The most common type of sleep disorder. This condition may cause difficulty falling asleep, staying asleep, or awakening. Many people have experienced a period of transient insomnia for less than one week due to stress or environmental changes. If this persists, it becomes acute insomnia (less than one-month duration) or evolves into what specialists call chronic insomnia (more than one-month duration). There are several potential causes of chronic insomnia, including

- chronic pain or other physical illness
- shift work
- poor sleep habits
- consuming too much alcohol or caffeine
- certain medications
- certain psychiatric conditions

In primary insomnia, individual differences in brain function may result in an overactive alerting signal that continues long after a person would like to fall asleep. There are a variety of treatment options available if underlying health issues or environmental factors cannot be identified or changed. Treatments include

- biofeedback
- meditation

- cognitive-behavioral therapy for insomnia (CBT-I)

I already reviewed biofeedback and meditation in chapter 4. CBT-I is a psychological intervention that typically lasts 8–12 weeks. In CBT-I, a provider will perform a series of sleep assessments, ask you to complete a sleep diary, and work with the you in session to help change the way you sleep. CBT-I is a safe and effective means of managing chronic insomnia. This program can help you even if your sleep problems have a biological origin. The program does not use sleep medications but instead teaches you how to improve your sleep by changing your behavior. CBT-I includes

- relaxation training
- cognitive restructuring
- stimulus control

- sleep restriction
- sleep hygiene
- relapse prevention

People need to learn how to maintain what they've learned and prepare for a future flare-up. If a flare-up occurs, it is important that you do not sleep more during the day to compensate for sleep loss. In addition, you should restart stimulus control procedures and re-engage in sleep restriction if symptoms persist. There are five general areas that influence sleep hygiene:

1. **Circadian rhythms:** These rhythms influence when, how much, and how well people sleep. They can be altered by various factors, including naps, bedtime, exercise, and exposure to light. Some recommendations for improving sleep hygiene include maintaining a regular bedtime and awakening time (including on weekends), getting out of bed at the same time every day, exercising regularly (finishing a few hours before bedtime), avoiding naps, and going to bed only when sleepy.

2. **Age:** Aging also plays a role in sleep and sleep hygiene. There are many more nocturnal awakenings after people reach the age of 40.

3. **Psychological stressors:** It is beneficial for people to develop a pre-sleep ritual to break the connection between stress and bedtime. Relaxing rituals can include a warm bath or shower, aromatherapy, reading, listening to soothing music, drinking a warm glass of milk, and eating small portions of seeds and nuts, cheese, or soy. Of note, you should finish eating about two to three hours prior to your regular bedtime. You may also want to designate another time of the day to write down problems

and possible solutions instead of thinking of such things at bedtime. In addition, strenuous exercise during the day may promote better sleep, as long as it's at least three hours before bedtime.

4. **Substance use:** Many people rely on caffeine daily to function. Caffeine is a stimulant that causes people to be more energized, awake, and capable of sustaining intellectual activity. Caffeine can be consumed in coffee, tea, soda, energy drinks, and chocolate and takes 15 to 45 minutes to reach its maximum effect. Caffeine can stay in the body for up to 14 hours and can lead to disturbed sleep. You should avoid consuming caffeinated beverages within 6 hours of your regular bedtime. Tobacco contains nicotine that causes stimulation and almost immediately increases energy and alertness affecting sleep. An indirect public health problem related to tobacco is accidental fires. If you cannot give up smoking, it is recommended that you discontinue smoking 2 hours before bedtime. Alcohol initially can help people become sedated, making it easier for them to fall asleep. The downside to alcohol is that it causes arousal 2 to 3 hours after it is metabolized and cleared. You should discontinue use of alcohol within 2 hours of bedtime. Many prescription medications and OTC medicines can cause sleep problems. Illicit drugs also can negatively affect sleep. Smoking marijuana tends to reduce REM sleep, MDMA has arousing properties, and cocaine both increases wakefulness and suppresses REM sleep.

5. **Sleep Environment:** You should also consider environment factors, such as temperature and noise. Your sleeping environment should be relatively cool, dark, quiet, and comfortable. You should be sleeping on a comfortable mattress and pillow. Be aware that you should be flipping your mattress regularly and you will need to update your mattress after four years. The bedroom is to be used only for sleep and sex, and having a computer, tablet, cell phone, or TV on in the bedroom is discouraged.

Sexual Health

According to the World Health Organization, sexual health is a state of biopsychosocial well-being in relation to sexuality. Sexual health it is not merely the absence of dysfunction. Most studies of the sexual activity of people who suffer from chronic pain report worsening in sexual health, including frequency and quality. No relationship has been found between pain severity, duration, frequency, and sexual functioning. A relationship has been found between disability status, age, and psychological variables (depression and anxiety) and domains of sexual response cycle (desire, arousal, and orgasm). In order to make a comprehensive diagnosis and a recommendation for treatment, providers must include sexual function in their medical review of patients with chronic pain.

Sexual dysfunctions are highly prevalent, affecting about 43% of women and 31% of men. Sexual desire disorders have been reported in approximately 30% of women and 15% of men. Pain or even the fear of pain can decrease desire, making people uninterested in sex. Sexual arousal disorders have been reported in 10% to 20% of men and women. Sometimes chronic pain may hinder or block sexual excitement, causing the man to have trouble achieving an erection or a woman to have trouble secreting vaginal fluid. If a person becomes excited, but the act causes pain, the excitement may be reversed. Orgasmic disorders have been reported in 10% to 15% of women. Inability to have an orgasm can sometimes be related to lack of knowledge about how women orgasm and the appropriate clitoral stimulation that may be needed for women to reach climax. Reportedly, men on average reach climax in 2.8 minutes, while women on average achieve orgasm in 13 minutes. In other cases, the inability to reach orgasm may be related to either neuropathy or may be medication induced. Pain medications may delay time to climax/orgasm or completely stop the climax from occurring in men and women as they alter sensation. The pain sensation itself can also prevent people from reaching climax during sex. About 30% of men may also suffer from premature ejaculation, especially younger populations. Finally, sexual pain disorders have been reported in 10% to 15% of women and less than 5% of men. Sexual pain disorders in women typically occur in the vulvar area and most commonly are related to hormonal deficiency and/or a state of abnormally high muscle tension. Sexual pain disorders in men typically involve groin pain and may be related to infection or trauma to the groin area.

Sexual health also requires a positive and respectful approach to sexuality and sexual relationships that are consensual among adults. Sometimes chronic pain can alter the way people feel about themselves. It may cause them to have low self-esteem or to feel depressed. These feelings can interfere with sexual desire. Some people find that chronic pain strains their relationships with their sexual partners because of their mood. As a result, they tend not to be very attentive to their partners, which may cause their partners to become impatient and feel differently toward them. Despite the pairing, the relationship is the key to sexuality. If the relationship is in conflict, then the pairing may need some conflict resolution. There are different sexual needs when one person in a pairing has an illness, such as chronic pain. People are taught to take responsibility for their own sexual satisfaction, and worry less about holding their partner accountable. Thus, good communication is essential and the couple may need psychological counseling or enrichment programming.

Chronic pain may hinder a person's ability to move freely, and thus, limit the positions they can get into to have sex. Sometimes chronic pain requires partners change the sexual positions or acts they've grown accustomed to in order to find a position that doesn't cause pain. There are several different sexual positions with recommendations to prevent people from hurting their back. These recommendations may generalize to all pairings if modified to reflect the sex of those involved. Note that aids are used during the sexual act such as pillows, and body posture such as knee and hip alignment remains important. Again, it's important that pairings spend time touching, kissing, and hugging as forms of foreplay after sex and even when they don't have sex but want to express affection towards one another.

If a person with chronic pain continues to report sexual dysfunction, a referral to a sexual health clinic may be beneficial. Sexual health clinics may provide different services, including

- sex education
- evaluation and treatment for sexual dysfunction
- contraception (condoms and birth control)
- physical examinations and labs (hormone levels)
- sexually transmitted infection testing and treatment
- vaccinations (hepatitis A/B and human papillomavirus)

Sexual health providers will also evaluate each person to determine what factors or drugs may be affecting their sexual function. There are several factors that affect sexual dysfunction, including

- chronic medical illness (diabetes, cardiovascular, and hypertension)
- psychiatric illness (depression and bipolar disorder)
- trauma or surgery (Peyronie's disease, prostatectomy, and radiotherapy)
- modifiable risk factors (smoking tobacco, using alcohol, sedentary lifestyle, and obesity)
- medications (antihypertensives, antidepressants, antihistamines)
- illicit drugs (opiates, cocaine, methadone)

Sexual healthcare professionals can also provide several different treatment options, including

- coaching
- sensate focus (discovering erogenous zones through non-genital stimulation)
- vacuum devices
- intracavernosal injections
- pharmacological agents
- herbs

Vocational Rehabilitation

Pain is the number-one cause of adult disability in the United States. Approximately 13% of the total workforce reported experiencing a loss in productive time during a two-week period of employment due to pain. Workers who were missing from productive time due to pain lost a mean of 4.6 hours/week. The majority of the lost productive time (77%) was explained by reduced performance while at work and not work absence. A 2010 report by the Institute of Medicine indicated that the annual value of lost productivity ranged between $297 billion and $335 billion. The value of lost productivity was based on three estimates, including days of work missed, hours of work lost, and lower wages. For many people, employment is an essential part of identity. Work helps people

- gain a sense of pride and self-satisfaction
- earn money to cover bills and pay for activities during leisure time
- expand social networks
- develop new skills
- improve general mood and health

Research has shown that work is beneficial, while unemployment is associated with poorer physical health, mental health, and well-being. Work can be therapeutic and can reverse the adverse health effects of unemployment among many disabled people, people with common health problems, and social security beneficiaries. Thus, more and more attention is being paid to preventing disability and promoting return to work in pain management.

Vocational rehabilitation programs have been developed for people with chronic diseases. They consist of a systematic assessment of the problems at work and the development of individual solutions. The aims of vocational rehabilitation are to improve psychosocial skills and/or implement work accommodations. They use several different methods, including

- education
- assessment
- counselling
- training
- role playing

The most important outcome measures of vocational rehabilitation are

- employment status
- actions to arrange work accommodations
- psychosocial measures (self-efficacy and social competence)

Demographic, job-related, and psychological factors should be emphasized in the evaluation of vocational potential and the assessment of disability in people with pain. Jobs should be safe and accommodating for sickness and disability. Keep in mind that the beneficial effects of work outweigh the risks of work, the harmful effects of long-term unemployment, or prolonged sickness absence. There is some evidence that interventions that train people in requesting accommodations and feel self-confident to deal with problems are successful. Psycho-socio-demographic variables (sex and beliefs in vocational return) have also been found to be powerful overall predictors of failures. They are better predictors of vocational rehabilitation outcomes and superior to the signs and symptoms recorded by physicians. There is strong scientific evidence for vocational rehabilitation for musculoskeletal conditions.

The evidence suggests that effective vocational rehabilitation depends on work-focused healthcare and accommodating workplaces. They are interdependent and must be coordinated with the person in pain. The concept of early intervention is central to vocational rehabilitation—the longer you are off work, the greater the obstacles to returning. In the first six weeks or so, most people with common health problems can be helped to return to work. They can be helped by employers by following a few basic steps, including

- Identifying people after about 6 weeks' sickness absence
- Directing them to appropriate help
- Ensuring the content and standards of the interventions provided

Only 20% of people receiving incapacity benefits for more than six months will return to work in the following five years. For people who are out of work more than six months and on benefits, vocational rehabilitation needs to be reinforced by education. The education is about the value of work for health and recovery and integrated with management skills. For claimants with mental health problems and for long-term benefit recipients, these efforts may include a work-focused interview. This interview will help identify links between functional abilities and task demands in the workplace.

Past research studies have identified musculoskeletal disorders and contributions from psychiatric conditions as the most common causes for long-term unemployment. There are several other reasons a person may have been out of work for an extended period of time, including

- a lack of incentive to return to work
- previous claims for benefits have been denied
- accustomed to being off work
- negative impact on work ability due to demands on the body
- ineffective management of pain at work
- history of being punished at work due to pain

- perception that exposure to the employer, colleagues, or other aspects of work will lead to relapse

Potential responses to this information may include addressing

- job-related fears and dissatisfaction
- fears of re-injury
- psychosocial barriers to return to work
- adversarial relationships between employer and employee
- workplace accommodations that may be barriers

There is strong evidence that suggests that work disability duration is significantly reduced by work accommodation offers. There are a multitude of accommodations to consider, including

1. allowing use of paid or unpaid leave for medical treatment
2. providing self-paced workload or the ability to modify one's schedule
3. providing support for maintaining concentration
4. allowing for frequent breaks
5. dividing large assignments into smaller tasks and steps
6. scheduling regular meetings with the supervisor to determine goals and address concerns
7. using organizers, calendars, and daily reminders
8. setting clear expectations of the person's responsibilities and consequences for not meeting them
9. establishing long and short-term goals
10. providing praise and positive reinforcement

Past research has suggested adopting the traditional disability paradigm in the design of work rehabilitation programs for workers with mental health problems. There are special accommodations that can be considered for people with mental health and addiction concerns, including

1. referring them to counseling or employee assistance programs
2. providing structure
3. allowing a flexible schedule for counseling or attendance to AA/NA meetings
4. not mandating job-related social functions with exposure to triggers
5. providing healthy and sober working environment
6. avoiding references to drugs and alcohol
7. encouraging employees to use company-sponsored health programs

Vocational rehabilitation efforts for claimants with mental health problems and for long-term benefit recipients may also include support services, such as developing a resume and interviewing skills. Innovative programming that includes obtaining and supervising work trials to help claimants with mental health problems and for long-term benefit recipients acclimate to the routine of work may also be offered along with return to work credit, or financial support.

The following is a list by state of available organizations that can assist you in job search activities and gaining employment.

A Quick Resource Guide

Alabama: http://www.rehab.alabama.gov/individuals-and-families/vocational -rehabilitation-service-general
Alaska: http://www.labor.state.ak.us/dvr/home.htm
Arizona: http://www.azdes.gov/RSA
Arkansas: http://www.arsinfo.org
California: http://www.rehab.cahwnet.gov
Colorado: http://www.dvrcolorado.com
Connecticut: http://www.brs.state.ct.us
Delaware: https://joblink.delaware.gov/ada/r
Florida: http://www.rehabworks.org
Georgia: http://gvra.georgia.gov
Hawaii: http://www.hawaiivr.org
Idaho: http://www.vr.idaho.gov
Illinois: https://www.dhs.state.il.us/page.aspx?item=29737
Indiana: http://www.in.gov/fssa/2328.htm
Iowa: http://www.ivrs.iowa.gov
Kansas: http://www.dcf.ks.gov/services/ees/Pages/Work/WorkProgram.aspx
Kentucky: http://ovr.ky.gov
Louisiana: http://wwwprd.doa.louisiana.gov/laservices/publicpages/servicedetail .cfm?service_id=2857
Maine: http://www.maine.gov/rehab
Maryland: http://www.dors.state.md.us
Massachusetts: http://www.mass.gov/eohhs/gov/departments/mrc
Michigan: http://www.michigan.gov/mdcd/0,1607,7-122-25392---,00.html
Minnesota: http://www.deed.state.mn.us/rehab
Mississippi: http://www.mdrs.ms.gov/VocationalRehab/Pages/default.aspx
Missouri: http://dese.mo.gov/vr
Montana: http://www.dphhs.mt.gov/dsd/vrs/index.shtml
Nebraska: http://www.vr.nebraska.gov
Nevada: http://detr.state.nv.us/rehab/reh_vorh.htm
New Hampshire: http://education.nh.gov/career/vocational
New Jersey: http://jobs4jersey.com/jobs4jersey/jobseekers/disable/index.html
New Mexico: http://www.dvrgetsjobs.com
New York: http://www.acces.nysed.gov/vr
North Carolina: http://www.ncdhhs.gov/dvrs
North Dakota: http://www.nd.gov/dhs/dvr/index.html
Ohio: http://ood.ohio.gov
Oklahoma: http://www.okrehab.org
Oregon: http://www.oregon.gov/DHS/vr
Pennsylvania: http://www.portal.state.pa.us/portal/server.pt/community/vocational _rehabilitation/10356
Rhode Island: http://www.ors.state.ri.us

South Carolina: http://www.scvrd.net
South Dakota: http://dhs.sd.gov/drs/vocrehab/vr.aspx
Tennessee: http://www.tennessee.gov/humanserv/rehab/vrs.html
Texas: http://www.dars.state.tx.us
Utah: http://www.usor.utah.gov
Vermont: http://vocrehab.vermont.gov
Virginia: http://www.vadrs.org
Washington: http://www.dshs.wa.gov/dvr
West Virginia: http://www.wvdrs.org
Wisconsin: http://dwd.wisconsin.gov/dvr
Wyoming: http://wyomingworkforce.org/job-seekers-and-workers/vocational
-rehabilitation

Spirituality & Religion

Healthcare systems in the United States have begun implementing a new medical care model that is more aligned with a biopsychosocial–spiritual approach to health. The renewed biopsychosocial–spiritual approach emphasizes the person's responsibility for self-management and should include education, wellness principles, and sound interventions. Such a comprehensive approach must be used in chronic pain management. Health professionals should serve their patients' needs as a "whole," including their mind, body, and spirit. Chronic pain can be considered a disruption in biological relationships that in turn affects all the other relational aspects of a person. Spirituality concerns a person's relationship with transcendence, or "whole"-ness. Scholars suggest that many people would like health professionals to attend to their spiritual needs. However, healthcare providers must be cautious and avoid preaching.

The topic of "spiritual healing" or "spiritual acts" is riddled with controversy due to its religious implications. Certain religious groups may believe that these practices are condemned in the Holy Bible, New International Version. For example, Deuteronomy 18 (v. 10–11) states, "Let no one be found among you who sacrifices their son or daughter in the fire, who practices divination or sorcery, interprets omens, engages in witchcraft, or casts spells, or who is a medium or spiritist or who consults the dead." Others shy away from these practices because they equate spirituality with religion. Spiritual healing is largely nondenominational, and traditional religious faith is not a prerequisite for therapy.

As noted, pain management should treat people as a whole—their mind, body, and spirit. But how do you define spirit? In athletics, spirit may mean excitement or passion. In sacred texts, it denotes the breath of life. In modern times, it connotes meaning or purpose. *Meaning* is a sense of beliefs or values. *Purpose* is a sense of direction or aim. Spirituality is the aspect of humanity that refers to the way people seek and express meaning and purpose. It is the way they experience their connectedness to the moment, to self, to others, to nature, and to the significant or sacred. A chronic illness, however, can cause people to question their meaning and purpose in life. The medical literature suggests that it is important to discuss spirituality because such efforts

- increase overall satisfaction with health care
- improves quality of life
- increases clinical effectiveness in pain management

In 1946, Viktor Frankl described in *Man's Search for Meaning* how concentration camp inmates' pain and suffering eased once they found meaning and purpose in their lives. Spirituality matters to many people who experience pain. In addition, people may struggle to make sense of their pain experience. Those who struggle with their spirituality are at risk for inadequate pain management. The relationship between spirituality and healing can be traced back into antiquity. Historically, the priest, the physician, and the psychologist were the same person in some societies. The advent of scientific medicine in the mid-nineteenth century separated the body from the mind and spirit nearly completely. A century later, the direct interrelationship between the body and mind became firmly established. Over the past several decades, there has been a broad revival of interest in spiritual healing and health. Spirituality may have analgesic properties, inoculate against depression and suicide, add psychosocial support, decrease risky behaviors, provide a means for community integration, and give meaning or "existential coherence."

There are several practices people in pain can engage in to increase their spirituality. Prayer is the simplest form of self-care and has been found to be the most common medical intervention used in the United States. Prayer is a reverent petition made to an object of worship. The three largest faith groups in this country are Christianity, Judaism, and Islam. Perhaps providers should encourage their patients from those faiths to use prayer as a form of pain management. Meditation is a devotional exercise of or leading to contemplation. It is perhaps a more secular or neo-sacred approach or alternative to the process of prayer. See chapter 4 for more information about the practice of meditation. A simpler method of introspection may be for people to read words of hope and inspiration from such resources as

- *Our Daily Bread*
- *Portals of Prayer*
- Mahatma Gandhi quotes
- *Guideposts*

People may present with barriers to everyday practice of these methods, including sedation from medications, relaxation wariness, unwillingness to look beyond the self, and difficulties in setting boundaries.

Chaplain services have been integrated in most healthcare systems. They are available to facilitate spiritual healing by providing chapel worship, sacraments and rites, memorial services, inpatient hospitalization visits, and other types of spiritual care. At times, chaplain services may not provide exactly what the person seeks. In such cases, chaplain services may be able to provide alternative choices via a network of other clergy and spiritual leaders within the community.

A Quick Prayer Guide

Religion	Sample Prayer
Christian	"O God, the Source of all health and healing, so fill my heart with faith that with calm expectancy I may receive Your power to help me in this time of my need. By Your grace and mercy through Jesus Christ, Our Lord and Savior, forgive my sin, heal my spirit, mind and body, and be present with me. Guide my doctors, nurses and other staff by Your counsel so they will have skill, wisdom and ability to help me. Amen."
Jewish	"O God, Source of life and all of its blessings. You are the healer of the sick. I turn to you in my time of trouble and pray for strength from you. Give me faith to rely on Your love and power to hope that I shall be well. Bless with Your wisdom the efforts of all who work to restore me to health. Heal me and I shall be healed; save me and I shall be saved. Amen."
Muslim	"O Allah, remove the hardship, O Lord of mankind, grant cure, for You are the Healer. There is no cure but from You, a cure which leaves no illness behind."

A Closer Look

What do you mean by the term "spirituality"?

Spirituality is a framework or an umbrella term used to define a set of experiences that are very personal to each individual. Researchers have linked the awe we feel when touched by the beauty of nature, art, and spirituality with lower levels of proinflammatory cytokines. These proteins signal the immune system to work harder. There are several other ways people who suffer from chronic pain can integrate spiritual healing in their lives, including

• reconciling with themselves or others

- joining spiritual support groups
- becoming one with nature
- reading sacred spiritual passages or performing rituals
- engaging in movement programs
- journaling or starting other reflective practices
- participating in the arts

Religion   Nature
          Art

Traditional Healers

Perhaps some of you may be interested in seeking spiritual healing from traditional healers. A traditional healer is someone who employs any one of a number of ancient medical practices that are based on indigenous theories, beliefs, and experiences handed down from generation to generation. The methods employed by each type of traditional healer have evolved to reflect the different philosophical backgrounds and cultural origins of the healer. There are several options to consider in for your treatment plan, including

- **Botanica:** A traditional healer who supplies healing products, sometimes associated with spiritual interventions.
- **Curandero:** A type of traditional folk healer originally found in Latin America. Curanderos specialize in treating illness through the use of supernatural forces, herbal remedies, and other natural medicines.
- **Espiritista:** A traditional healer who assesses a person's condition and recommends herbs and religious amulets to improve physical or mental health or to help overcome a personal problem.
- **Hierbero or Yerbera:** A traditional healer or practitioner with knowledge of the medicinal qualities of plants.
- **Native American Healer/Medicine Man:** A traditional healer who uses information from the spirit world in order to benefit the community. People see Native American healers for a variety of reasons, especially to find relief or a cure from illness or to find spiritual guidance.
- **Shaman:** A traditional healer who is said to act as a medium between the invisible spiritual world and the physical world. Most gain knowledge

through contact with the spiritual world and use the information to perform tasks such as divination, influencing natural events, and healing the sick or injured.

- **Sobador:** A traditional healer who uses massage and rub techniques in order to treat people.

A Closer Look

What gets in the way of these practices?

People may present with barriers to these everyday practices. It can be a difficult path. Consider, as an example, "The Wall," by Gloria J. Evans, a modern parable that details the consequences of surrounding ourselves with protective walls that isolate us from love and fellowship.

A simple measure of privacy can gradually become more complex and fortified due to fear, anger, jealousy, resentment, self-pity, and indifference. These stressful experiences can lead to people being unable to live their lives and becoming deconditioned, which will lead to more pain. In order to move forward, the wall needs to be deconstructed by encouraging people to seek meaning, pride, joy, love, forgiveness, and healthy relationships.

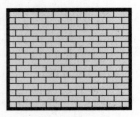

Recreation

I often call recreation therapy the "crown jewel" of comprehensive pain management. Recreation therapy is a treatment service designed to restore, remediate, and rehabilitate a person's level of functioning and independence in life activities. According to the American Therapeutic Recreation Association, the goals are to promote health and to reduce limitations that restrict participation in life. The word "recreation" defines the role of the recreation therapist—to "re-create" a means of activity. Intervention areas vary widely and are based upon your interests, including

- exercise programming (see chapter 5)
- adaptive sports
- leisure education
- creative arts (music and fine art)

Unfortunately, research has shown that providers tend to give recreation therapies a lower endorsement when compared to other pain management modalities. This is due to their low practical and theoretical exposure to this type of intervention. Theoretically, recreation therapy could be thought of as an adult version of child "play therapy."

Adapted sports: These are based on existing able-bodied sports, modified to meet the needs of persons with a disability. Many sports are practiced by persons with a disability outside formal sports movements, such as the Paralympics or Warrior Games. Some examples of adapted sports include

- bowling
- golf
- equine therapy
- archery
- scuba diving
- skiing

Leisure education: This focuses on three subcategories: sports and recreation, tourism, and leisure. In recreation, tourism is considered travel for leisure and is of limited duration. Tourism is commonly associated with travel within the community for the purpose of reintegration. Examples of tourism may include

- trips to local park districts
- attractions and tours
- free community events
- entertainment (theatre or sports events)

Leisure, or "free time," is time spent away from other responsibilities including activities of daily living. Leisure activities include a very broad range of activities, including the arts and other hobbies.

Creative Arts: A background in music or fine arts is not always necessary. Creative arts therapists make these mediums accessible for everyone. There are various reasons for the integration of these forms of therapy in complementary, supportive pain management programs, including their

1. enhancement in activity level and creative capacity as a healing source
2. stimulation of positive emotional experience
3. communication and social interaction
4. facilitation in coping
5. stimulation of imaginative experience and awareness
6. promotion of suggestions

Music therapists primarily help people improve their health by using music experiences such as drum circles and singing karaoke. Research suggests that drumming serves as a distraction from pain and promotes the production of endorphins and endogenous opiates. Past studies also suggest that active singing may have some benefits in terms of active coping. Past research has also shown that music can increase the effectiveness of medical therapies and can be used as an adjuvant with other pain-management programs. The definition of art therapy varies depending on its focus. The art-making process can be therapeutic in and of itself, or it can be used in combination with other therapies. The purpose of art therapy is essentially one of healing. In art therapy, any type of visual art and art medium can be employed within the therapeutic process, including

- painting
- drawing
- sculpting
- photography
- digital art

One study found that people explored their narrative and experience and allowed providers to gain understanding about their journey using art. Art therapy stands in contrast with other kinds of creative arts therapies, such as dance or theater.

Lifestyle Management Summary

Chronic diseases are among the most common, costly, and preventable of all health problems according to the CDC. The incidence of heart disease, diabetes, and cancer combined is lower than that of chronic pain. In the United States, 86% of all healthcare spending in 2010 was for people with one or more chronic diseases. Alarming projections suggest future generations may have shorter, less healthy lives. Healthcare costs in the United States will rise to $4 trillion, the equivalent of four Iraq wars in a single year if current trends continue. Specific health risk behaviors cause much of the illness, suffering, and early death related to chronic diseases and conditions. The roadmap to health is simple:

- Eat real food
- Practice self-love
- Imagine yourself well
- Get sufficient sleep
- Incorporate movement into your life

Thus, the solution to our nation's pain crisis does not seem complicated.

Conclusion

In the previous chapters, I reviewed all the options currently available for the treatment of chronic pain. Chapter 6 was the last chapter, and it reviewed lifestyle imbalances that are affected by chronic pain, including nutrition, functional medicine, weight loss, sleep hygiene, sexual health, vocational rehabilitation, spirituality and religion, traditional healers, and recreation. The following chapters will shift the focus away from treatment and towards ways to empower people with chronic pain and review different coping strategies.

References

Ajzen I, Fishbein M. (1980). Understanding attitudes and predicting social behavior. Englewood Cliffs, NJ: Prentice-Hall.

Alaska Sleep Clinic. Alaska sleep education center. 2015. http://www.alaskasleep.com/blog/problems-solutions-sleeping-cpap-mask. Accessed July 3, 2015.

Althof S. (2006). Sexual therapy in the age of pharmacotherapy. *Annual Review of Sex Research*, 116–132.

American College of Preventative Medicine. (2016). Lifestyle Medicine Initiative. Available at: http://www.acpm.org/page/ LifestyleMedicine. Accessed June 1, 2016.

American College of Sports Medicine. (2013). ACSM's Guidelines for Exercise Testing and Prescription (9th ed.) LWW.

American Osteopathic Association (2016). Available at http://www.osteopathic.org/inside-aoa/about/leadership/ Pages/tenets-of-osteopathic-medicine.aspx. Accessed September 9, 2016.

American Psychiatric Association. *Diagnostic and Statistical Manual of Mental Disorders*. 5th ed. Washington, DC: American Psychiatric Association; 2013.

American Sleep Apnea Association. OSA treatment options. 2015. http://www.sleepapnea.org/treat/treatment-options.html. Accessed July 3, 2015.

American Therapeutic Recreation Association. Promoting health and wellness services. Available at: https://www.atra-online.com/. Accessed May 14, 2015.

Anandacoomarasamy A, Fransen M, March L. (2009). Obesity and the musculoskeletal system. *Current Opinion in Rheumatology*, 21, 71–77.

Anxiety and Depression Association of America. Screenings for depression, anxiety, and PTSD. Available at: http://www.adaa.org/ Accessed June 2, 2015.

Bernatzkya G, Prescha M, Anderson M, et al. (2011). Emotional foundations of music as a non-pharmacological pain management tool in modern medicine. *Neuroscience and Biobehavioral Reviews*, 35, 1989–1999.

Better Sleep Council. Physical performance and sleep. http://bettersleep.org/better-sleep/healthy-sleep/physical-performance-sleep. Accessed June 22, 2015.

Block J, DeSalvo K, Fisher W. (2003). Are physicians equipped to address the obesity epidemic? Knowledge and attitudes of internal medicine residents. *Preventive Medicine*, 36, 669–675.

Breivik H, Collett B, Ventafridda V, Cohen R, Gallacher D. Survey of chronic pain in Europe: prevalence, impact on daily life, and treatment. *Eur J Pain*. 2006; 10(4):287–333.

Briand C, Durand M, St-Arnaud L, et al. (2007). Work and mental health: Learning from return-to-work rehabilitation programs designed for workers with musculoskeletal disorders. *International Journal of Law and Psychiatry*, 30, 444–457.

Brody S. (2010). The relative health benefits of different sexual activities. *The Journal of Sexual Medicine*, 7, 1336–1361.

Brown AC, Gluten senstitivity: problems of an emerging condition separate from celiac disease. *Expert Rev Gastroenterol Hepatol* 6 (2012): 43–55.

Brown C, Barner J, Richards K, et al. Patterns of complementary and alternative medicine use in African Americans. *J Altern Complement Med*. 2007; 13(7):751–758.

Brown C, Richardson C. (2006). Nurses' in the multi-professional pain team: A study of attitudes, beliefs and treatment endorsements. *European Journal of Pain*, 10, 13–22.

Centers for Disease Control. (2016). Available at: http://www.cdc.gov/chronicdisease/overview/index.htm. Accessed June 1, 2016.

Christensen R, Astrup A, Bliddal H. (2005). Weight loss: The treatment of choice for knee osteoarthritis? A randomized trial. *Osteoarthritis Cartilage*, 13, 20–27.

Clayton A, Montejo A. (2006). Major depressive disorder, antidepressants, and sexual dysfunction. *Journal of Clinical Psychiatry*, 67, S33–S37.

Cleveland Clinic. Drug and alcohol related sleep disorders. 2013.http://my.clevelandclinic.org/services/neurological_institute/sleep-disorders-center/disorders-conditions/hic-drug-and-alcohol-related-sleep-disorders. Accessed July 3, 2015.

Clinical Nutrition: A Functional Approach. 2nd ed. Levin JS et al. Gig Harbor, Washington: Institute for Functional Medicine, 2004.

Cohen S, Mount B, Bruera E, et al. Validity of the McGill Quality of Life Questionnaire in the palliative care setting: A multi-centre Canadian study demonstrating the importance of the existential domain. *Palliat Med.* 1997; 11(1):3–20.

Colbert J, Jangi S. (2013). Training physicians to manage obesity- Back to the drawing board. *New England Journal of Medicine*, 369, 1389–1391.

Cooper Z, Doll H, Hawker D, et al. (2010). Testing a new cognitive behavioral treatment for obesity: A randomized controlled trial with three-year follow-up. *Behavior Research & Therapy*, 48, 706–713.

Craig K. Biopsychosocial approach in pain management: A case study. 2012. Available at: http://www.nilpain.org/webstorage/webstorage5/Biopsychosocial%20approach%20in%20pain%20management%20-%20a%20case%20study%20hypothesis.pdf. Accessed March 12, 2013.

Daenen L, Varkey E, Kellmann M, et al. (2014). Exercise, not to exercise, or how to exercise in patients with chronic pain? Applying science to practice. Clinical Journal of Pain. Accessed May 18, 2015.

Daily Devotions on Portals of Prayer. 2013. Available at: http://sites.cph.org/portals. Accessed June 27, 2013.

Department for Work and Pensions. (2002). *Pathways to work: Helping people into employment*. London: Stationery Office.

Derby C, Mohr B, Goldstein I, et al. (2000). Modifiable risk factors and erectile dysfunction: Can lifestyle changes modify risk? *Urology*, 56, 302–306.

Donini L, Savina C, Castellaneta E, et al. (2009). Multidisciplinary approach to obesity. *Eating & Weight Disorders*, 14, 23–32.

Edwards D. (2004). *Art therapy*. London: Sage Publications.

Eklund M. (1992). Chronic pain and vocational rehabilitation: A multifactorial analysis of symptoms, signs, and psycho-socio-demographics. *Journal of Occupational Rehabilitation*, 2, 53–66.

Engel G. The need for a new medical model: A challenge for biomedicine. *Science.* 1977; 196:129–136.

Estimate from the Millken Institute report. (2016). An Unhealthy America: The economic impact of chronic disease. Available at: http://www.chronicdiseaseimpact.com. Accessed June 1, 2016.

Eustice C, Eustice R. Gout foods: Avoiding purine-rich foods. Your Guide to Arthritis. Available at: http://www.afhaz.com/ images/dietgout.pdf. Accessed May 6, 2015.

Evans G. *The Wall: A Parable*. New York, NY: W Publishing Group; 1977.

Fasano A. Leaky gut and autoimmune diseases. *Clin Rev Allergy Immunol* 42 (2012): 71–78.

Franche R, Cullen K, Clarke J, et al. (2005). Workplace-based return-to-work interventions: A systematic review of the quantitative literature. *Journal of Occupational Rehabilitation*, 15, 607–631.

Frankl V. *Man's Search for Meaning*. Boston, MA: Beacon Press; 2006.

Frederick B. (1980). *Body mechanics: Instructional manual: A guide for therapists*. Lynwood, WA: Banfac Enterprises.

Gearhardt AN, Davis C, Kuschner R, Brownwell KD. The addiction potential of hyperpalatable foods. *Curr Drug Abuse Rev* 4 (2011): 140–45.

Goldstein I, Krane, R. (1983). Drug-induced sexual dysfunction. *World Journal of Urology*, 1, 239–243.

Guideposts Magazine. 2013. Available at: http://www.guideposts. org /. Accessed June 27, 2013.

Haba-Rubio J, Krieger J. Evaluation instruments for sleep disorders: a brief history of polysomnography and sleep medicine. Accessed July 3, 2015.

HealthAliciousNess.Com. Top 10 foods highest in tryptophan. 2015. http://www.healthaliciousness.com/articles/high-tryptophan-foods.php. Accessed July 3, 2015.

Healthline. Central Sleep Apnea: Causes. 2015. http://www.healthline.com/health/sleep/central-sleep-apnea#Causes2. Accessed July 3, 2015.

Heiman J, Talley D, Bailen J, et al. (2007). Sexual function and satisfaction in heterosexual couples when men are administered sildenafil citrate (Viagra) for erectile dysfunction: A multicenter, randomized, double-blind, placebo-controlled trial. *British Journal of Obstetrics and Gynecology*, 114, 437–447.

Henare D, Hocking C, Smythe L. (2003). Chronic pain: Gaining understanding through the use of art. *British Journal of Occupational Therapy*, 66, 511–518.

Henderson M, Glozier N, Elliot K. (2005). Long term sickness absence is caused by common conditions and needs managing. *British Medical Journal*, 330, 802–803.

Holy Bible, New International Version®, 1973, Biblica, Inc. Permission from Zondervan.

Hooper M. (2006). Tending to the musculoskeletal problems of obesity. *Cleveland Clinic Journal of Medicine*, 73, 839–845.

Hyman M. The last diet you will ever need. Huffington Post, 6/3/12. Available at: http://www.huffingtonpost.com/dr-mark-hyman/food-industry_b_1559920.html. Accessed May 6, 2015.

Hyman, M. A. (2010). The failure or risk factor treatment for primary prevention of chronic disease. *Alternative Therapy in Health and Medicine*, 16, 60–63.

Institute of Medicine of the National Academies Report. (2011). *Relieving pain in America: A blueprint for transforming prevention, care, education, and research*. The National Academies Press, Washington DC.

Institute of Medicine. Caffeine for the sustainment of mental task performance: formulations for military operations. http://www.iom.edu/reports/2001/caffeine-for-the-sustainment-of-mental-task-performance-formulations-for-military-operations.aspx. Accessed July 3, 2015.

Janke E, Collins A, Kozak A. (2007). Overview of the relationship between pain and obesity: What do we know? Where do we go next? *Journal of Rehabilitation & Research Development*, 44, 245–262.

Jarow J, Lowe F. (1997). Penile trauma: An etiologic factor in Peyronie's disease and erectile dysfunction. *The Journal of Urology*, 158, 1388–1390.

Jones J, Huxtable C, Hodgson J, et al. (2003). *Self-reported work-related illness in 2001/2002.* London: HSE.

Kaartinen K, Lammi K, Hypen M, et al. (2000). Vegan diet alleviates fibromyalgia symptoms. *Scandinavian Journal of Rheumatology*, 29, 308–313.

Kelley D. (2001). Modulation of human immune and inflammatory responses by dietary fatty acids. *Nutrition*, 17, 669–673.

Kenny D, Faunce G. (2004). The impact of group singing on mood, coping and perceived pain in chronic pain patients attending a multidisciplinary pain clinic. *Journal of Music Therapy*, 41, 241–258.

Kjekdsen-Kragh J. (1999). Rheumatoid arthritis treated with vegetarian diets. *American Journal of Clinical Nutrition*, 70, 594S–600S.

Konlian C. (1998). Aquatic therapy: Making a wave in the treatment of low back injuries. Orthopedic Nursing: PDF only. Available at: http://journals.lww.com/orthopaedicnursing/ Abstract/1999/01000/ Aquatic_Therapy__Making_a_Wave_in_the_Treatment_of.4.aspx.

Lauman E, Paik A, Rosen R. (1999). Sexual dysfunction in the United States: Prevalence and predictors. *Journal of the American Medical Association*, 281, 537–544.

Lim J, Tchai E, Jang S. (2010). Effectiveness of aquatic exercise for obese patients with knee osteoarthritis: A randomized controlled trial. *PM&R: The Journal of Injury, Function, & Rehabilitation*, 2, 723–731.

Mahatma Gandhi quotes. 2013. Available at: http://www.brainy quote.com/quotes/authors/m/ mahatma _gandhi.html. Accessed June 27, 2013.

Maruta T, Osborne D. (1978). Sexual activity in chronic pain patients. *Psychosomatics*, 19, 531–537.

Masters W, Johnson V. (1970). *Human sexual inadequacy.* Boston: MA. Little, Brown.

Mayank G, Gautam D, Priyanka A, et al. Depression-sleep disturbance-chronic pain syndrome. *Indian J Pain.* 2014; 28(3):177–183.

Melnick T, Soares B, Nasello A. (2008). The effectiveness of psychological interventions for the treatment of erectile dysfunction: Systematic review and meta-analysis, including comparisons to sildenafil treatment, intracavernosal injections and vacuum devices. *Journal of Sexual Medicine*, 5, 2562–2574.

Merck Manual Consumer Version. Alcohol: drug use and abuse. 2015. https://www.merckmanuals.com /home/special-subjects/drug-use-and-abuse/alcohol. Accessed July 3, 2015

Milhous R, Haugh L, Frymoyer J, et al. (1989). Determinants of vocational disability in patients with low back pain. *Archives of Physical Medicine and Rehabilitation*, 70, 589–593.

Miller W, Rollnick S. (2002). *Motivational interviewing: Preparing people to change.* Guilford press.

Misic P, Arandjelovic D, Stanojkovic S, et al. (2010). Music therapy. *European Psychiatry*, 1, 839.

Monga T, Tan G, Ostermann H, et al. (1998). Sexuality and sexual adjustment of patients with chronic pain. *Disability and Rehabilitation*, 20, 317–329.

Mornhinweg G, Voignier R. (1995). Holistic Nursing Interventions. Orthopedic Nursing, PDF only. Available at: http://journals.lww.com/orthopaedicnursing/Abstract/1995/07000/Holistic_Nursing _Interventions.4.aspx.

Müller-Busch H. (1991). Art therapy in chronic pain. *Der Schmerz*, 5, 115–121.

Nancarrow S, Booth A, Ariss S, et al. (2013). Ten principles of good interdisciplinary team work. *Human Resources for Health*, 11, 19.

National Heart, Lung, and Blood Institute. Portion Distortion. Available at: http://www.nhlbi.nih.gov /health/educational/ wecan/eat-right/portion-distortion.htm. Accessed May 11, 2015.

National Institute of Health. NIH state-of-the-science conference statement on manifestations and management of chronic insomnia in adults. *NIH Consens State Sci Statements.* 2005; 22(2):1–30.

National Institute of Neurological Disorders and Stroke. Restless legs syndrome fact sheet. 2015. http:// www.ninds.nih.gov/ disorders/restless_legs/detail_restless_legs.htm. Accessed July 3, 2015.

National Sleep Foundation. Cognitive behavioral therapy for insomnia. 2015. http://sleepfoundation.org /sleep-news/cognitive-behavioral-therapy-insomnia?page=0%2C0. Accessed July 3, 2015.

National Sleep Foundation. Recommended Sleep. 2015. http://sleepfoundation.org/how-sleep-works/how -much-sleep-do-we-really-need. Accessed July 3, 2015.

National Sleep Foundation. What causes insomnia? 2014. http://sleepfoundation.org/insomnia/content /what-causes-insomnia. Accessed July 3, 2015.

Neuman W. Nutrition Plate Unveiled, Replacing Food Pyramid. New York Times, 6/2/11. Available at: http://www.nytimes.com/ 2011/06/03/business/03plate.html?_r=0. Accessed May 6, 2015.

Olshansky, S. J., Passaro, D. J., Hershow, R. C., Layden, J., Carnes, B., ... Ludwig, D. S. (2005). A potential decline in life expectancy in the United States in the 21st century. *The New England Journal of Medicine*, 352, 1138–1145.

PAIRS Foundation. Helping veterans strengthen most significant relationships. 2012. Available at: http://veterans.pairs.com/. Accessed March 12, 2013.

Peltonen M, Lindroos A, Torgerson J. (2003). Musculoskeletal pain in the obese: A comparison with a general population and long-term changes after conventional and surgical obesity treatment. *Pain*, 104, 549–557.

Pietrzykowska N. Obesity Action Coalition. Benefits of 5-10 percent weight-loss. Accessed May 7, 2015.

Puchalski C, Ferrell B, Virani R, et al. Improving the quality of spiritual care as a dimension of palliative care: The report of the Consensus Conference. *J Palliat Med*. 2009; 12(10): 885–904.

Puchalski C. Making healthcare whole: Integrating spirituality into patient care (GWish). Available at: https://smhs.gwu.edu/staticfile/SMHS/Graduate%20Medical%20Education/Feb%202011%20Spirituality%20in%20Medicine.pdf. Accessed October 5, 2012.

Quesenberry C, Caan B, Jacobson A. (1998). Obesity, health services use, and health care costs among members of a health maintenance organization. *Archives of Internal Medicine*, 158, 466–472.

Ray L, Lipton R, Zimmerman M, et al. (2011). Mechanisms of association between obesity and chronic pain in the elderly. *Pain*, 152, 53–59.

Rosen H. Patient information: Calcium and vitamin D for bone health (Beyond the Basics). Available at: http://www.uptodate.com/contents/calcium-and-vitamin-d-for-bone-health-beyond-the-basics?source=see_link. Accessed May 6, 2015.

Rosner F. Religion and Medicine. 2011. Available at: http://www.pensgard.com/nutrition/18_Religion.htm. Accessed October 5, 2012.

Ruser C, Sanders L, Brescia G, et al. (2005). Identification and management of overweight and obesity by internal medicine residents. *Journal of General Internal Medicine*, 20, 1139–1141.

Santrock, J. *A Topical Approach to Human Life-span Development (3rd ed)*. St. Louis, MO: McGraw-Hill; 2007.

Schatz C. Mindfulness meditation improves connections in the brain. *Harvard Women's Health Watch*. April 08, 2011.

Schierenbeck T, Riemann D, Berger M, Hornyak M. Effect of illicit recreational drugs upon sleep: Cocaine, ecstasy and marijuana. *Sleep Med Rev*. 2008; 12(5):381–389.

Sellinger J, Clark E, Shulman M, et al. (2010). The moderating effect of obesity on cognitive–behavioral pain treatment outcomes. *Pain Medicine*, 11, 1381–1390.

Selvin E, Burnett A, Platz E. (2007). Prevalence and risk factors for erectile dysfunction in the US. *The American Journal of Medicine*, 120, 151–157.

Sjogren K, Fugl-Meyer A. (1981). Chronic back pain and sexuality. *International Rehabilitation Medicine*, 3, 19–25.

Somers T, Wren A, Keefe F. (2011). Understanding chronic pain in older adults: Abdominal fat is where it is at. *Pain*, 152, 8–9.

Stewart W, Ricci J, Chee E, et al. (2003). Lost productive time and cost due to common pain conditions in the U.S. workforce. *Journal of the American Medical Association*, 290, 2443–2454.

Substance Abuse and Mental Health Services Administration. Office of Applied Studies. Results from the 2013 National Survey on Drug Use and Health: Summary of national findings. Accessed on July 3, 2015.

Tennant F. A Diet for Patients with Chronic Pain. Practical Pain Management, 7/1/11. Available at: http://www.practicalpainmanagement.com/treatments/complementary/diet-patients-chronic-pain. Accessed May 6, 2015.

Textbook of Functional Medicine. Gig Harbor, Washington: Institute for Functional Medicine, 2010

The Institute of Functional Medicine. (2016). About functional medicine. Available at: https://www.functionalmedicine.org/What_is_Functional_Medicine/AboutFM. Accessed June 1, 2016.

The Wahls Protocol: A radical new way to treat all chronic autoimmune conditions using paleo principles. Wahls T. Penguin Group, 2014.

Thong S. (2007). Redefining the tools of art therapy. *Art Therapy: Journal of the American Art Therapy Association*, 24, 52–58.

Thought of the Day from Our Daily Bread. 2013. Available at: http://odb.org/. Accessed June 27, 2013.

University of Kentucky. Chronic low back pain and how it may affect sexuality. 2003. Available at: http://www.drcharlesblum.com/Patient%20Information/Chronic%20Low%20Back%20Pain%20and%20How%20it%20May%20Effect%20Sexuality%20August%202003.pdf. Accessed August 17, 2012.

Unruh A. Spirituality and Nature. 2004. Available at: http://www.umb.no/statisk/helse/unruh.pdf. Accessed October 5, 2012.

Unruh A. Spirituality, religion, and pain. *Can J Nurs Res*. 2007; 39(2):66–86.

US Department of Veterans Affairs. John D. Dingell VA Medical Center: Sleep Center Education. http:// www.detroit.va.gov/Detroit/services/sleepcenter_educ_3col.asp. Accessed July 3, 2015.

Varekamp I, Verbeek J, van Dijk F. (2006). How can we help employees with chronic diseases to stay at work? *International Archives of Occupational and Environmental Health*, 80, 87–97.

Waddell G, Aylward M, Sawney P. (2002). *Back pain, incapacity for work, and social security benefits: An international literature review and analysis.* London: Royal Society of Medicine Press.

Waddell G, Burton A, Kendall N (2008). *Vocational rehabilitation: What works, for whom, and when?* London: TSO.

Waddell G, Burton A. (2006). Is work good for your health and well-being? Department for Work and Pensions, HM Government and The Stationery Office. London: TSO.

WebMD. Sleep Disorders Health Center. Cognitive behavioral treatments for sleep problems. 2015. http:// www.webmd.com/ sleep-disorders/behavioral-treatments. Accessed July 3, 2015.

Weil A. Dr. Weil's Anti-Inflammatory Diet. Available at: http://www.drweil.com/drw/u/ART02012/anti -inflammatory-diet. Accessed May 6, 2015.

Williams J, Meltzer D, Arora V, et al. Attention to inpatients' religious and spiritual concerns: Predictors and association with patient satisfaction. *J Gen Intern Med.* 2011; 26(11):1265–1271.

Winkelman M. (2000). *Shamanism: The neural ecology of consciousness and healing.* Westport, Connecticut: Bergin & Garvey.

World Health Organization (WHO). Reproductive health. Available at: http://www.who.int/topics /reproductive _health/en/. Accessed May 19, 2015.

Yunus M, Arslan S, Aldag J. (2002). Relationship between body mass index and fibromyalgia features. *Scandinavian Journal of Rheumatology*, 31, 27–31.

Chapter 7

Empowering Providers & People with Chronic Pain

The purpose of this chapter is to help people in their efforts to lead healthier lives. Several skills will be reviewed in this chapter, including how to select treatments, communicate successfully, set realistic goals, deal with difficult behaviors, instill hope, and set boundaries. It is important that people who suffer from chronic pain remain engaged in the process of improving their care and maintain their role as the primary investors in their health care system.

Questions for the Reader to Ponder

By the end of this chapter, you should be able to answer the following questions:

1. Which pain management modality is the best to use?
2. Which factors are common across therapies and have been found to contribute more to treatment outcomes than specific interventions?
3. What challenges the therapeutic relationship?
4. How can improving my communication skills improve my pain?
5. How can I set appropriate boundaries?

Selecting Treatments

Often people who suffer from chronic pain and other health professionals will ask me how to determine the best treatment modality to use. You may have come to the conclusion after reviewing chapters 3–6 that most treatments will offer a mild to moderate reduction of pain. The current evidence provides little support for choosing one approach over another. Some of you might find this conclusion to be discouraging. However, there are other things to consider in your treatment, including:

- Pain-related factors
  » Type and intensity of pain
  » Physical and cognitive abilities
  » Coexisting symptoms

- Individual-related factors
  » Previous experiences and expectations for outcome
  » Cultural and spiritual influences
  » Patient preferences and coping styles

- Environmental factors
  » Involvement of friends and family

A Closer Look

How long does it take to obtain real control over my pain?

It is important to remember that pain management takes time. It takes 50% of people with moderate pain at least 6 months to reach a point of real control after adopting a multidisciplinary approach. The more severe their pain, the longer it will take to get it under control. A successful treatment goal should be a 40–60% reduction in pain over a 6-month period. Remember, most treatment modalities reviewed in chapters 3–6 offer a mild to moderate reduction of pain:

- 30–60%   physical fitness
- 30–60%   CBT/mindfulness
- 30–50%   antidepressants/anticonvulsants
- 30–50%   opioid medications
- 10%   acupuncture

What is interesting is that people will report that treatment modalities may be of some benefit for pain management when combined with other treatments. However, the percentage of improvement may not be additive, but rather complementary.

So, if you report your pain to be a "10," the most you should expect is a reduction of 4–6 points. At best, your pain will reduce to about a "4–6." If your pain is a "5," then you should expect a reduction of about 2–3 points, which brings you to a low score of "2–3." Remember, that is not bad, considering that most people walk around with anywhere between a "2–3" in their pain level.

Goldilocks Effect

People with chronic pain and their providers try different treatments until they find something that works, a phenomenon referred to as the "Goldilocks effect." The name is derived from the children's tale of *The Three Bears*. In the story, Goldilocks wanders far from home and stumbles upon the house of the three bears. She tries all their chairs, tastes all their porridge, and lies in all their beds. Goldilocks finds the baby bear's the most suitable for her in all three cases.

Unfortunately, people try different options and do not give them enough time to see if they work. Then they move on to the next treatment. This affects the success rate of that type of treatment. If you wanted to study the success rate of acupuncture, you would need to find a sample of people with chronic pain who have had pain for more than five years to be representative. It would be hard to find people to do that study who have not already tried other treatments. This would affect whether people found improvement with acupuncture alone without considering past treatments. This is why research has shown that the overall success of treatment for chronic pain remains inconsistent and fairly poor. The practice of psychotherapy confronted a similar issue in the past. The field of pain management may be able to glean insight from the psychological research in "common factors."

Common Factors

References to the concept of common factors began as early as 1936. Research studies at that time found that all psychotherapies were successful—a conclusion later termed the "dodo bird effect." This is a reference to the character from *Alice's Adventures in Wonderland*. In the original story, the dodo bird is the character who proposes that everyone run a caucus race. The participants were to run in different patterns in order to get dry after a swim. He says this so that everyone wins and "all must have prizes." Hans Eysenck wrote one of the classic papers in the history of psychology in 1952. He announced that psychotherapy did not lead to improved patient outcomes. In response, mental health providers began conducting research to explain the psychotherapy process and outcomes. A summary of the review of research has shown that psychotherapy is undeniably successful as a treatment. Two important findings have been noted from those analyses. First, the effect of psychotherapy did not change despite how conservative or rigorous the research study. In addition, all the different types of psychotherapy had the same effects. These conclusions led to the distinction of two possible means of psychotherapeutic change: "specific" and "nonspecific" effects. Specific effects were associated with unique interventions to certain therapy approaches. Nonspecific effects were linked with common factors of the clinical encounter.

Factors common across therapies have been found to contribute more to treatment outcomes than effects associated with specific technical interventions. A summary of the review of research then summarized psychotherapy outcome research and reduced the factors into four areas:

- Patient factors—the characteristics of the patient and his/her environment—were found to explain 40% of the change in outcomes.
- Therapeutic relationship—the characteristics of the patient and the provider that facilitate change and are present regardless of the type of intervention—were found to explain 30% of the change in outcomes.
- Expectancy/placebo/hope—improvements that result from the patient and provider's belief that treatment is successful—were found to explain 15% of the change in outcomes.
- Techniques/models—such as the traditional, holistic, and Eastern practices discussed previously—were found to explain 15% of the change in outcomes.

This research later inspired a book titled *The Great Psychotherapy Debate*. In that book, the author concluded that nonspecific effects were responsible for more than 4 times the amount of change in treatment outcomes across various interventions. Using models developed in other professions to inform inquiry in another field is appropriate. There is some precedence in literature, specifically in physical medicine and rehabilitation. Is it possible that these nonspecific effects are responsible for some amount of change in treatment outcomes in pain management?

Common factors speak to pain management being an art form in addition to a science. From a psychotherapy perspective, specific interventions discussed previously will not be fully successful without adding the other common factors. There is evidence to suggest that these same common factors may be responsible for general effects in pain management.

Manumea Effect

Research studies in pain management have concluded that the diverse treatment interventions currently available all appear to be successful. I propose this verdict to be termed the "manumea effect," referencing Samoa's endangered tooth-billed pigeon. The manumea is similar to the dodo bird, which is appropriate since it is a relative of this famously extinct bird. It is also cryptic, and almost invisible in its nature. Even though a common factors model in pain management is not fully developed, such a model should be considered in order to further advance knowledge and practice in pain medicine.

Patient Factors

Patient factors include several different themes, such as social support, faith, and strengths/abilities. It would appear from the current research that treatment outcomes were better when the patient

- was employed, which affected recovery.
- was motivated to manage pain.
- perceived having social support.
- believed in a spiritual power greater than themselves.
- did not experience any recent/daily life stressors.
- had positive beliefs and used coping strategies.
- felt they had control over outcomes in their lives.
- felt they had control over their pain.
- was able to recover and remained positive.
- was engaged in activities that were purposeful.
- had a readiness to change.
- had high treatment outcome expectations.

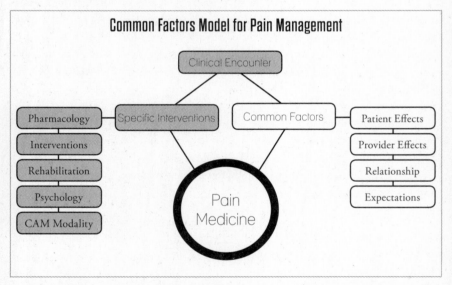

According to the research, it is important for you to maintain your employment while in the process of recovery. If you are not employed, I would recommend that you work with a vocational rehabilitation counselor. See chapter 6 for more information.

Some people may react to that recommendation by saying "I'm not motivated." People tend to get motivated when they hit rock bottom. Unfortunately, motivation for some of us comes from fear or anxiety. The good news is that you can change that by

- educating yourself about the positive effects of certain foods, social connections, and exercises (as outlined in chapter 6).
- doing small increments of your tasks.
- becoming aware of your thoughts.
- being truthful to yourself.
- tapping into gratitude for the things you can do.

Remember, this is about changing your mindset in order to witness some success.

Everything today is viewed as not being our fault but is rather the result of a disease, addiction, or chemical imbalance. As a society, we need to stop being a victim and start taking control of our lives. You must first accept the fact that you do not have control of anyone else except yourself. The good news is that you can take control of your life by

- asking questions, doing research, and watching others.
- asking yourself, "What do I want? What is my desired outcome?"
- coming up with two or more potential solutions to the problem.
- taking action.
- looking back at the effects of your actions—"What's working? What isn't?"
- learning from the feedback you get.
- changing your efforts.

There is a lot of negativity in this world, and it can be easy to fall into it. In fact, when we wake up in the morning our brains are already set to think negatively! I have learned that there are things we can do to stay positive and live a positive life. The good news is that you can bring more positivity into your life by

- seeing the positive in negative situations. "What is this bad situation trying to teach me?"
- having a positive living and social environment (including the virtual world).
- having positive self-talk.
- becoming more thankful for the things you have.
- continuing to improve yourself.
- living each day with purpose.

Therapeutic Relationship

The therapeutic relationship, also therapeutic alliance, helping alliance, or working alliance, is a psychotherapy common factor. It was identified by Grencavage and Norcross in 1990 and has been validated by strong research support. Research on the power of the therapeutic relationship now reflects more than 1,000 research findings. It has been found to predict treatment loyalty, agreement, and outcome across a range of patient diagnoses and treatment settings. Therapeutic relationship factors include several different themes, such as the patient-provider relationship and encouragement/instruction. It would appear from the current research that

- patient-provider relationship is associated with outcome.
- provider empathy plays a crucial role in pain treatment.
- providers who are warm are more successful.
- people are more satisfied when they perceive they are respected by providers.
- people's suffering may be affected by recognition of real pain.
- people need to learn to accept chronic pain.
- patient encouragement and instruction decreases pain and increases satisfaction.
- the communication process influences self-management of pain.

The patient-provider relationship is the key mediator between perceived helpfulness and patient satisfaction. In reality, the right to effective pain management comes with shared responsibilities between the person who suffers from pain and their provider. However, these relationships can be challenged. People who suffer from chronic pain and providers have opposing attitudes and goals. One person tries to control the other. Someone asserts control and the other person is left to concede. This leads to tension, power struggles, increased feelings of stigmatization, distrust, and discomfort in treatment. People who suffer from pain want their pain to be legitimized, feel questioned, and try to be more credible. They perceive providers as lacking in empathy, doubting their pain is real, and being influenced by stereotypes. Providers want to avoid feeling powerless—there is no cure, no improvement, and no consolation prize, at times. Providers report being more concerned about other urgent health conditions, looking for objectivity within a subjective condition, and not taking ample time to build relationship of trust. Providers do not engage in more shared medical decision making because they believe it will increase their workload. They are reluctant to engage with people who appear to lack comprehension. Some providers will even discontinue treatment if the person in pain engages in complementary and integrative health treatments over standard medical care.

People who have rewarding relationships with their health care providers have better outcomes and are less likely to seek assistance from other sources. This reduces the risk of conflicting treatment plans and further confusion. The success of this working alliance often determines whether a person with chronic pain will adopt self-management strategies. Essential elements of a healthy therapeutic relationship include

- Compassion
- Clear expectations
- Adequate explanations by the provider
- Active participation and involvement in decision-making by the person in pain

For Providers

Communication Can Bridge the Gap

People with chronic pain and providers may benefit from communication training. Successful communication is one of the most important life skills. We don't usually put a lot of effort into this skillset. Increased attention on communication has been proposed as a way to improve the therapeutic relationship. There are seven pathways to better health through communication:

1. Increased access to care
2. Greater patient knowledge and shared understanding
3. Higher quality medical decisions
4. Enhanced therapeutic alliances
5. Increased social support
6. Patient agency and empowerment
7. Better management of emotions

Providers can improve communication by investing in the beginning of their relationship with the person who suffers from pain. It is important that they create a bond and let the person tell their story. Providers may want to ask the person in pain for their ideas, requests, and how they see pain impacting their life. They want to be aware of their own reactions to the person suffering and be open to that person's emotions. Providers must also invest in the end of their relationship by leaving the person in pain with needed education, a diagnosis, and engaging them in shared medical decision making.

There are five essential components to good communication, which include

1. Really listening
2. Expressing empathy

A Closer Look

How do I really listen?

It is important for you to distinguish what listening is. Listening is *not*

- Ordering, directing, or commanding
- Warning or threatening
- Giving advice, making suggestions, or providing solutions
- Persuading with logic, arguing, or lecturing
- Moralizing, preaching, or telling people their duty
- Judging, criticizing, disagreeing, or blaming
- Agreeing, approving, or praising
- Shaming, ridiculing, or name calling
- Interpreting or analyzing
- Reassuring, sympathizing, or consoling
- Questioning or probing
- Withdrawing, distracting, humoring, or changing the subject

People often confuse empathy for sympathy. Empathy is the ability to understand and share the feelings of another person. It is seeking the world through their eyes. It is your ability to understand what they are saying and see it from their point of view. We need to see the other person as a human being. Someone who is valuable in their own right. Someone who we need to approach without judgement. We need to get in touch with our own emotions in order to truly connect with another person's feelings. A common reason to skip this element of empathy is that we don't have our own emotions sorted out.

You also need to communicate understanding. This helps the other person feel like they are being understood, that they are seen, and heard. If you don't know what to say, say, "Tell me more about it." There are several ways you can improve your empathy skills:

- Reading good literature
- Studying history
- Being present with a friend at work

There are also communication skills you can use to communicate your empathy. One way to do this is by using affirmations. Affirmations are statements that recognize the other person's strengths. They assist in building a bond but are only effective when they are genuine. Affirmations often involve expressing behaviors or concerns differently and as evidence of positive qualities. Affirmations are a key element in supporting self-efficacy.

A Closer Look

What number do you see?

Empathy is the ability to see the world through someone else's eyes. Look at the number below. What number you see depends on from which perspective you have. For example, if you look at the number from your far left, you may see the number 9. If you look at the number from the far right, you may see the number 6. However, you are viewing the same number from a different perspective.

3. Being concise

Summaries are one way to help you be concise. Summaries are a special type of reflection where you recap what has occurred in all or part of an appointment. Summaries communicate interest and understanding and call attention to important elements of the discussion. They may be used to shift attention or direction. Providers can use summaries to help the person in pain prepare to move forward. They can also be used to highlight the person's readiness to change.

4. Asking questions and reflecting

Asking questions and reflecting can also help with communication between you and the other person. Although closed-ended questions have their place, open-ended questions create forward momentum. Open-ended questions are not easily answered with a "yes/no" or short answer. Open-ended questions invite explanation and thinking more deeply about an issue. Reflection refers to the person "reflecting" back the other person's words. This is done to allow the other person to hear for themselves what they have said and evaluate the logic or reasoning behind their own statements.

5. Watching your body language

A Closer Look

What does my body language say?

Your body language can communicate different things to other people. It is important that you are aware of what your body is communicating and whether that is your intention. The following is a list of behaviors and what they say about you:

- Fidgeting—conveys being nervous
- Looking up or looking around—a cue someone is lying
- Staring—can be interpreted as aggressive
- Failing to smile—can make people uncomfortable
- Stepping back when asking for a decision—conveys fear
- Standing with hands on hips—is an aggressive posture
- Checking phone or watch—says you want to be somewhere else
- Hands behind your back or in pockets—looks rigid and stiff
- Leaning back too much—comes off lazy or arrogant
- Leaning forward—can seem aggressive
- Breaking eye contact soon—seems untrustworthy or nervous
- Nodding too much—nod once and then try to remain still
- Pointing with your hands—feels aggressive
- Crossing your arms—you look defensive
- Steepling fingers or holding palms up—conveys weakness

For Providers

Setting Realistic Expectations

Expectancy factors include several different themes, such as expectations. It would appear that treatment outcomes are enhanced when

- people expect and believe treatment is potentially beneficial
- providers consider how placebo effects improve outcomes
- providers consider the person's potential to be noncompliant and relapse
- people are optimistic, have hope, or accept their pain
- people feel providers believe their pain is credible

There are expectations that people have of their providers, including that they

- be thoughtful and listen
- be empathetic and nonjudgmental
- do no harm and be competent

Providers also have expectations of their patients, including that they

- be open and honest
- be obedient and motivated to get better
- display gratitude and pleasure at improvement

The challenge that I give to you, whether you are the person in pain or the provider, is to ask yourself if you are meeting the expectations of the other person.

Dealing with Difficult Behaviors

People who suffer from pain at times are deemed difficult, and providers can also present with common failures. It is important to remember that there are no difficult people, just people with difficulties! So why are people deemed difficult? There are several different reasons, including that they have

- a history of being mistreated, robbed, or ignored
- personality conflicts
- social or financial problems
- a lack of trust, information, or communication
- cultural differences/language barriers
- cognitive impairment
- severe mental health/addiction concerns
- advantages that occur secondary to stated illness
- system concerns
- negative drug interaction

Providers also have common failures. They use jargon and avoid certain topics. They can offer too much information and assume the other person is understanding them. They forget that their patients may be afraid to assert themselves. They at times make jokes and ignore or are unaware of how this impacts the other person. Providers may fail to explain that they work at a teaching hospital and how their clinics function. Providers are also made to feel like a police officer, judge, or deal-maker, which they did not receive training for or wish to engage in.

A Closer Look

A word about personalities . . .

As children, I learned that different characters have different personalities. One way I learned this was through the books by A. A. Milne: *Winnie-the-Pooh* and the *House on Pooh Corner*. Let's test to see which character you are most familiar with. It's probably not the one you think! Which character is

1. Easy-going, carefree?
2. Predictable, neat, and orderly?
3. Despairing, downtrodden, and ever-depressed?
4. Anxiety-ridden, perpetually uncertain?
5. In denial and sees only the positive?

1. Tigger; 2. Rabbit; 3. Eeyore; 4. Piglet; 5. Pooh

Boundary Setting

It is apparent that pain management, in particular, requires appropriate boundary setting. This is crucial regardless of the treatment plan, in part because people often find it hard to identify potential disagreements in their relationships. Boundaries are simply rules or limits that individuals create to identify reasonable, safe, and permissible ways for others to behave around them and to determine how they'll respond when someone oversteps these boundaries.

A Closer Look

How do I know if I have difficulty setting boundaries?

People who have difficulties setting boundaries in their personal life will have problems setting boundaries in their professional lives. As yourself the following questions:

- Is it hard for you to say no or yes?
- Are you ok when others say no to you?
- Do you take on other people's problems or pain?
- Do you experience other people's problems or pain?
- Do you share personal information quickly or slowly?
- Is it hard for you to share anything?
- Do you tell people in your life what you want, what you need, and how you feel?
- Are you able to ask for help when you need it?
- Is someone hurting or disrespecting you?

Establishing appropriate boundaries is a skill that requires a lot of thought and practice. Yet many people have learned little about it in school or in clinical training. To master this skill, it is important to recognize that a boundary is not a threat or an attempt to control the behavior of others, and that setting appropriate limits will ultimately improve relationships with people. There are four steps involved in setting appropriate boundaries:

1. **Name** or describe the behavior that is unacceptable
2. **Express** what you need or expect from the other person
3. **Decide** what you will do if they do not respect the boundaries you've established
4. **Validate** your actions by recognizing that setting boundaries is important work and that your rights are important

Many people feel uncomfortable during the boundary-setting process. Remember that setting boundaries is important work (Step 4: Validate). When reasonable limits are placed on a person and they continue to step beyond those limits, it is imperative that you maintain the boundary and be consistent with your message. Sometimes, saying "No" is the appropriate treatment! Therefore, efforts should be shifted from simply rejection to redirection—pointing people towards healthier options.

Instilling Hope

The instillation of hope offers a path back to a sense of possibility in our lives when almost all seems lost. It's a chance to look forward and wonder what might be over the horizon. Hope gives you strength and fuel to keep putting one foot in front of the other. Sometimes instilling hope is about looking backwards. You may want to ask yourself the following questions:

- What has hope looked like in your life?
- If you could see a photograph of hope, what might you see?
- How have you instilled, invoked, or strengthened hope in your life?
- What has undermined hope?
- How have you protected hope?
- What did it feel like for you to hope? Daring? Foolish? Reckless? Painful? Strong?
- How did hope impact how you saw yourself?
- Has hope formed a solid foundation for you?

The Last Patient Story

Sometimes, what people may want may not be what they need and saying "No" may be the therapy. Early on in my career, I worked with a young returning veteran who had come to the pain clinic asking to have his opioids refilled. I remember discussing the risks and benefits of the opioid medication with him and educating him about the comprehensive approach to pain management. In this case, the patient seemed to be in agreement with our plan because he nodded his head. I later got a call from his private psychologist, who argued with me. He questioned why I was discouraging the patient to use his pain medications. I had to re-educate that provider about the multidisciplinary approach and the need for him to provide a consistent message to the patient. The psychologist did relay that message to the patient. The patient was appropriately weaned off the opiates in the pain clinic, but then he moved away to another state and we lost contact. About a year later, I was at a concert venue and this individual approached me and thanked me for what we had done for him. He admitted being addicted to the opioid medication at that time, and said we provided the boundaries for him to stop taking them—boundaries he could not hold himself. He still had pain but was maintaining his employment at the concert venue and was living his life the best way he could.

Revisiting Patient Stories

Throughout chapters 3–5, cases were presented and a question was raised after each type of treatment was reviewed. In chapter 3, I had three case examples for the three traditional approaches being reviewed.

When discussing medications . . .

I introduced a 68-year-old male who went to a pain clinic for the first-time reporting neck and lower back pain. He had suffered from pain since the 1960s after several car accidents. He discussed at length all the various opioids he had been on throughout the years with his doctor. He also shared that he had repeatedly been able to "wean himself off" of opioids in the past. He was in the pain clinic hoping that a 30-day supply of fentanyl patches could be prescribed. He expected that the opioid should help considering his history.

In this example, you should consider the impact of the medications being used. However, you should also consider the impact of the expectations of the person and any other patient factors. In this example, there was also the potential that the individual was suffering from an opioid use disorder.

When discussing pain interventions . . .

I introduced a 69-year-old male who returned to the pain clinic after having a medial blanch block for arthritis in his joints of his spine about six months ago. The patient reported that he continues to have relief from the MBB, which is similar to the outcomes he has had in the past with other injections. The relief from the MBB should have only lasted a couple of hours.

Again, you should consider the impact of the pain intervention. However, you should also consider the impact of the expectations of the person and the therapeutic relationship. The patient had multiple injections/procedures in the past and had built a relationship with the pain clinic team.

When discussing physical medicine and rehabilitation . . .

I introduced a 68-year-old male suffering from early stages of Parkinson's disease who went to the pain clinic in a motorized wheelchair accompanied by his son. Since he had been coming to the pain clinic, he had physical and occupational therapy at home. The patient and his son felt this had made a significant improvement in pain, strength, and coordination. The patient had exhausted the 12 sessions covered by his insurance. He was now requesting further visits at home if it can get approved due to barriers in his son's social situation.

The patient in this example was struggling with his independence—he mobilized with a wheelchair and was accompanied by his son. Physical therapy exercises have been shown to be successful but require that he continue them independently. Continuing to offer these services at home may continue the dependence and may be affecting the outcome.

In chapter 4, I had a case example for the holistic approaches being reviewed.

When discussing psychological interventions . . .

I introduced a 58-year-old female who went to the pain clinic diagnosed with pseudogout and fibromyalgia in a wheelchair and cast on her right knee. She noted that she "hurt her knee so people would pay attention" (to her verbal complaints). She completed a course of treatment including cognitive-behavioral therapy for pain and acceptance and commitment therapy and seemed to be coping with her pain better. Every time she saw her provider, she exclaimed, "There is my favorite doctor," and went in for a hug.

There are clear patient factors present in this case, including self-harm (she hurt her knee to prove she was in pain). She also appeared to have developed a strong therapeutic relationship with her favorite doctor.

In chapter 5, there was a case example for the complementary and integrative health approaches being reviewed.

When discussing complementary and integrative health . . .

I introduced a 62-year-old female who went to the pain clinic for about a year and tried all the different modalities available without any relief. The patient had a history of multiple traumas and had suffered two strokes. The current provider introduced her to a nurse who was similar characteristically to her and who had been trained in healing touch. The patient returned a month later and noted that the healing touch was the only thing that had worked for her and that she enjoyed working with the nurse.

In this example, one should consider the impact of the CIH approach. However, one should also consider the impact of the therapeutic relationship with that provider—a nurse who is similar to her. She may have been more comfortable with this particular provider due to their similar interests and her history of traumas. There is also the possibility that she had hoped this technique would help since it was referred to her by the pain clinic team.

Conclusion

Chapter 7 reviews ways in which to empower providers and people who suffer from chronic pain. The final chapter reviews different types of coping strategies that can be used by people who suffer from chronic pain and provides who may suffer from burnout. I start with a discussion comparing active versus passive coping and then review different treatment plans for different pain conditions. I end the chapter with strategies to cope with chronic pain that you can implement into your daily practice.

References

Alamo M, Moral R, Pérula de Torres L. Evaluation of a patient-centered approach in generalized musculoskeletal chronic pain/fibromyalgia patients in primary care. *Patient Educ Couns*. 2002; 48:23–31.

Andrews G, Harvey R. Does psychotherapy benefit neurotic patients? *Arch Gen Psych*. 1981; 38:1203–1208.

Armon C, Argoff C, Samuels J, et al. Assessment: use of epidural steroid injections to treat radicular lumbosacral pain: a report of the Therapeutics and Technology Assessment Subcommittee of the American Academy of Neurology. *Neurology*. 2007; 68:723–729.

Arnold L, Keck P, Welge J. Antidepressant treatment of fibromyalgia: a meta-analysis and review. *Psychosomatics*. 2000; 41:104–113.

Art of Manliness. (2010). Building Your Resiliency: Part III: Taking Control of Your Life. Available at: https://www.artofmanliness.com/2010/02/16/building-your-resiliency-part-iii-taking-control-of-your -life.

Attal N, Cruccu G, Baron R, et al. EFNS guidelines on the pharmacological treatment of neuropathic pain: 2010 revision. *Eur J Neurol*. 2010; 17:1113–e88.

Bair M, Matthias M, Nyland K, et al. Barriers and facilitators to chronic pain self-management: a qualitative study of primary care patients with comorbid musculoskeletal pain and depression. *Pain Med*. 2009; 10:1280–1290.

Bates M, Rankin-Hill L, Sanchez-Ayendez M. The effects of the cultural context of health care on treatment of and response to chronic pain and illness. *Soc Sci Med*. 1997; 45:1433–1447.

Bergman A, Matthias M, Coffing J, et al. Contrasting tensions between patients and PCPs in chronic pain management: A qualitative study. *Pain Med*.2013; 14:1689–1697.

Bordin E. The generalizability of the psychoanalytic concept of the working alliance. *Psychother Theory Res Pract*. 1979; 16:252–260.

Centers for Disease Control and Prevention. Drug overdose in the United States: fact sheet. 2013. Available at: www.cdc.gov/ homeandrecreationalsafety/overdose/facts.html.

Centers for Disease Control and Prevention. Guideline for prescribing opioids for chronic pain—United States 2016. Recommendations and Reports. 2016; 65:1.1–49.

Chou R, Atlas S, Stanos S, et al. Nonsurgical interventional therapies for low back pain. *Spine*. 2009; 34:1078–1093.

Chou R, Baisden J, Carragee E, et al. Surgery for low back pain: a review of the evidence for an American Pain Society Clinical Practice Guideline. *Spine*. 2009; 34:1094–1109.

Chou R, Loeser J, Owens D, et al. Interventional therapies, surgery, and interdisciplinary rehabilitation for low back pain. *Spine*. 2009; 34:1066–1077.

de Haes, H. & Teunissen, S. (2005). Communication in palliative care: a review of recent literature. *Current Opinion in Oncology*, 17, 345–350.

DeBerard M, Masters K, Colledge A, et al. Outcomes of posterolateral lumbar fusion in Utah patients receiving workers' compensation: a retrospective cohort study. *Spine*. 2001; 26:738–746.

Dixon K, Keefe F, Scipio C, et al. Psychological interventions for arthritis pain management in adults: a meta-analysis. *Health Psychol*. 2007; 26:241–250.

Dorflinger L, Kerns R, Auerbach S. Providers' roles in enhancing patients' adherence to pain self management. *Transl Behav Med*. 2013; 3:39–46.

Dworkin R, O'Connor A, Audette J, et al. Recommendations for the pharmacological management of neuropathic pain: an overview and literature update. *Mayo Clin Proc*. 2010; 85: S3–S14.

Epstein, R. & Street, R. (2007). *Patient-centered communication in cancer care: promoting healing and reducing suffering*. Bethesda, MD: National Cancer Institute.

Eysenck H. The effects of psychotherapy: an evaluation. *J Consult Psychol*. 1952; 16:319–324.

Finnerup N, Sindrup S, Jensen T. The evidence for pharmacological treatment of neuropathic pain. *Pain*. 2010; 150:573–581.

Frank JD, Frank JB. *Persuasion and Healing: A Comparative Study of Psychotherapy. 3rd ed*. Baltimore, MD: Johns Hopkins University Press; 1991.

Frantsve L, Kerns R. Patient-provider interactions in the management of chronic pain: Current findings within the context of shared medical decision making. *Pain Med*. 2007; 8:25–35.

Frey M, Manchikanti L, Benyamin R, et al. Spinal cord stimulation for patients with failed back surgery syndrome: a systematic review. *Pain Physician*. 2009; 12:379–397.

Friedly J, Nishio I, Bishop M, et al. The relationship between repeated epidural steroid injections and subsequent opioid use and lumbar surgery. *Arch Phys Med Rehabil*. 2008; 89:1011–1015.

Furlan A, Sandoval J, Mailis-Gagnon A, et al. Opioids for chronic noncancer pain: a meta-analysis of effectiveness and side effects. *Can Med Assoc J*. 2006; 174:1589–1594.

Gourlay DL, Heit HA, Almahrezi A. Universal precautions in pain medicine: A rational approach to the treatment of chronic pain. *Pain Med*. 2005; 6:107–112.

Gourlay DL, Heit HA. Pain and addiction: Managing risk through comprehensive care. *J Addict Dis*. 2008; 27:23–30.

Grant, M. (2013). Ten tips for communicating with a person suffering from chronic pain. Overcoming Pain Website.

Grencavage L, Norcross J. Where are the commonalities among the therapeutic common factors? *Prof Psychol Res Pr*. 1990; 21:372–378.

Gulbrandsen P, Madsen H, Benth J, et al. Health care providers communicate less well with patients with chronic low back pain: A study of encounters at a back pain clinic in Denmark. *Pain*. 2010; 150:458–461.

Guzman J, Esmail R, Karjalainen K, et al. Multidisciplinary rehabilitation for chronic low back pain: systematic review. *Brit Med J*. 2001; 322:1511–1516.

Hall J, Boswell M. Ethics, law, and pain management as a patient right. *Pain Physician*. 2009; 12:499–506.

Henschke N, Ostelo R, van Tulder M, et al. Behavioural treatment for chronic low-back pain. *Cochrane Database of Systematic Reviews*. 2010; 7.7.

Hoffman B, Papas R, Chatkoff D, et al. Meta-analysis of psychological interventions for chronic low back pain. *Health Psychol*. 2007; 26:1–9.

Hornberger J, Kumar K, Verhulst E, et al. Rechargeable spinal cord stimulation versus non-rechargeable system for patients with failed back surgery syndrome: a cost-consequences analysis. *Clin J Pain*. 2008; 24:244–252.

Hubble M, Duncan B, Miller S. *The Heart and Soul of Change: What Works in Therapy*. American Psychological Association; 1999.

Inflexxion. Screener and Opioid Assessment for Patients with Pain (SOAPP). Available at: www.pain.edu .org/soapp.asp. Accessed February 10, 2014.

Ives T, Chelminski P, Hammett-Stabler C, et al. Predictors of opioid misuse in patients with chronic pain: A prospective cohort study. *BMC Health Serv Res*. 2006; 6:46.1–10.

Jensen M, Patterson D. Hypnotic treatment of chronic pain. *J Behav Med*. 2006; 29:95–124.

Keller A, Hayden J, Bombardier C, van Tulder M. (2007). Effect sizes of non-surgical treatments of non-specific low-back pain. *Euro Spine J*. 2007; 16:1776–1788.

Kroenke K, Krebs E, Bair M. Pharmacotherapy of chronic pain: a synthesis of recommendations from systematic reviews. *Gen Hosp Psychiatry*. 2009; 31:206–219.

Lambert M. Psychotherapy outcome research: implications for integrative and eclectic therapists. In: Norcross & Goldfried. *Handbook of Psychotherapy Integration. 1st ed*. New York: Basic Books; 1992.

Landman J, Dawes R. Psychotherapy outcome: Smith and Glass' conclusions stand up under scrutiny. *Am Psychol.* 1982; 37:504–516.

Lifestyle Inspire. (2017). 6 Ways to Bring Positivity You're your Life. Available at: http://www.lifestyleinspire.com/6-ways-to-bring-positivity-into-your-life.

Luijsterburg P, Verhagen A, Ostelo R, et al. Effectiveness of conservative treatments for the lumbosacral radicular syndrome: a systematic review. *Eur Spine J.* 2007; 16:881–899.

Manchikanti L. The growth of interventional pain management in the new millennium: a critical analysis of utilization in the Medicare population. *Pain Physician.* 2004; 7:465–482.

Mason L, Moore R, Edwards J, et al. Systematic review of efficacy of topical rubefacients containing salicylates for the treatment of acute and chronic pain. *Brit Med J.* 2004; 328(7446): 995.

Matthias M, Parpart A, Nyland K, et al. The patient-provider relationship in chronic pain care: providers' perspectives. *Pain Med.* 2010; 11:1688–1697.

Miciak M, Gross D, Joyce A. A review of the psychotherapeutic 'common factors' model and its application in physical therapy: the need to consider general effects in physical therapy practice. *Scand J Caring Sci.* 2011; 26:394–403.

Montgomery G, DuHamel K, Redd W. A meta-analysis of hypnotically induced analgesia: how effective is hypnosis? *Int J Clin Exp Hypn.* 2000; 48:138–153.

Morley S, Eccleston C, Williams A. Systematic review and meta-analysis of randomized controlled trials of cognitive behavior therapy and behavior therapy for chronic pain in adults, excluding headache. *Pain.* 1999; 80:1–13.

National Center for Complementary & Integrative Health (2017). *Complementary Health Approaches for Chronic Pain: What the Science Says.* Available at: https://nccih.nih.gov/health/providers/digest/chronic-pain-science.

Psychcentral. (2015). 5 Steps to Increase Motivation. Available at: https://psychcentral.com/blog/archives/2015/03/01/5-steps-to-increase-motivation.

Robeck I. Introduction: it's never too late to start all over again. Available at: www.painedu.org/articles_timely.asp?ArticleNumber=50.

Roelofs PD, Deyo RA, Koes BW, et al. Non-steroidal anti-inflammatory drugs for low back pain. *Cochrane Database Syst Rev.* 2008 Jan 23; (1).

Rosenzweig S. Some implicit common factors in diverse methods of psychotherapy. *Am J Orthopsy.* 1936; 6:412–415.

See S, Ginzburg R. Choosing a skeletal muscle relaxant. *Am Fam Phys.* 2008; 78:365–370.

Setting personal boundaries. Learning and Violence Web site. Available at: www.learningandviolence.net/violence/ disclosure/boundaries.pdf.

Shapiro D, Shapiro D. Meta-analysis of comparative therapy outcome studies: a replication and refinement. *Psychol Bull.* 1982; 92:581–604.

Singh G, Triadafilopoulos G. Epidemiology of NSAID induced gastrointestinal complications. *J Rheumatol Supp.* 1999; 56:18–24.

Smith M, Glass G. Meta-analysis of psychotherapy outcome studies. *Am Psychol.* 1977; 32:752–760.

Stein, T., Frankel, R., & Krupat, E. (2005). Enhancing clinician communication skills in a large healthcare organization: A longitudinal case study. *Patient Education & Counseling*, 58, 4–12.

Street R, Makoul G, Arora N, et al. How does communication heal? Pathways linking clinician-patient communication to health outcomes. *Patient Educ Couns.* 2009; 74:295–301.

Taylor R, Van Buyten J, Buchser E. Spinal cord stimulation for chronic back and leg pain and failed back surgery syndrome: a systematic review and analysis of prognostic factors. *Spine.* 2005; 30:152–160.

Townsend C, Rome J, Bruce B, et al. Interdisciplinary pain rehabilitation programs. In: Ebert MH, Kerns RD. *Behavioral and Psychopharmacological Pain Management.* New York, NY: Cambridge University Press;2011.

Turk D, Wilson H, Cahana A. Treatment of chronic noncancer pain. *Lancet.* 2011 ;377:2226–2235.

Turner J, Loeser J, Deyo R, et al. Spinal cord stimulation for patients with failed back surgery syndrome or complex regional pain syndrome: a systematic review of effectiveness and complications. *Pain.* 2004; 108:137–147.

Turner J, Sears J, Loeser J. Programmable intrathecal opioid delivery systems for chronic noncancer pain: a systematic review of effectiveness and complications. *Clin J Pain.* 2007; 23:180–195.

van Tulder M, Malmivaara A, Hayden J, et al. Statistical significance versus clinical importance: trials on exercise therapy for chronic low back pain as example. *Spine.* 2007; 32:1785–1790.

Verhaak P, Kerssens J, Dekker J, et al. Prevalence of chronic benign pain disorder among adults: a review of the literature. *Pain.* 1998; 77:231–239.

Vowles K, Thompson M. The patient-provider relationship in chronic pain. *Curr Pain Headache Rep.* 2012; 16:133–138.

Vroman K, Warner R, Chamberlain, K. Now let me tell you in my own words: narratives of acute and chronic low back pain. *Disabil Rehabil.* 2009; 31:976–987.

Walters G. Boundaries. Out of the Fog Web site. Available at: http://outofthefog.net/CommonNonBehaviors
/Boundaries.html.

Wampold B, Mondin G, Moody M, et al. A meta-analysis of outcome studies comparing bona fide psychotherapies: empiricially, "all must have prizes." *Psychol Bull.* 1997; 122:203–215.

Wampold B. *The Great Psychotherapy Debate: Models, Methods, and Findings.* 1st ed. Mahwah, NJ: Lawrence Erlbaum Associates Inc.; 2001.

Zgierska A, Miller M, Rabago D. Patient satisfaction, prescription drug abuse, and potential unintended consequences. *JAMA.* 2012; 307:1377–1378.

Chapter 8

Coping with Pain

Coping is the act of investing your own conscious effort to solve personal and interpersonal problems. The term generally refers to adaptive coping strategies which reduce stress. In contrast, maladaptive coping strategies may increase stress. The success of the coping effort depends on the individual, the type of stress, and the circumstances. Coping responses are partly controlled by your personality, but also partly by your social environment.

Questions for the Reader to Ponder

By the end of this chapter, you should be able to answer the following questions:

1. What are common characteristics of people who suffer from chronic pain?
2. What is the difference between active versus passive coping?
3. How are the biomedical and biopsychosocial models different?
4. How do you treat specific pain conditions?
5. What are some adaptive strategies for coping with pain?

Common Characteristics

People who suffer from chronic pain share specific characteristics in four areas:

- Attitudes and beliefs
- Behaviors
- Family & environment
- Compensation & work issues

Attitudes & Beliefs. An attitude is the way a person expresses or applies their beliefs and values. Some people who suffer from chronic pain believe that their pain must be gone completely before they can return to work. If they hold on to that belief and act accordingly, then they will never return to work. Remember, it is normal for people to have some level of pain (between 2 and 3 on the pain scale). Some people who suffer from chronic pain believe that work is harmful. I am going to share a secret with you. Having a job is actually pretty healthy! Of course, it will be more helpful if you engage in time-based activity pacing throughout the day as outlined in chapter 4.

A Closer Look

How is work actually healthy and helpful for pain?

When you are employed, you have to engage in a series of activities throughout the day that you would otherwise not have to do. You have to

- wake up at a certain time in the morning
- take a shower and get dressed
- prepare your breakfast and eat
- get to work either by driving, riding a bus/train, or maybe even walking
- socialize with others at your job
- be organized and have a plan
- engage in time management

And so on. All these activities are healthy and can help people cope with their pain.

Often, people with chronic pain may misinterpret bodily sensations as pain when in fact they are experiencing anxiety. This is covered in more detail in chapter 2. These sensations can lead people to believe that pain is uncontrollable. This belief may discourage people from even trying to manage their symptoms. I typically use a climate analogy to help explain to people their role in their pain. Remember, climate is what you expect and weather is what you get. We cannot control when its sunny or cloudy or when it rains or snows. This is similar to the idea that we cannot control when our pain flares up. We can control what we wear or what we do to adapt to the weather. We can carry an umbrella, wear a heavy coat, wear sunglasses, or run into a nearby shop to get out of the rain. This is similar to the idea that we can be active, eat healthy, relax, and sleep well to prepare for a pain flare-up. We need to take an active role in our pain management. When people with pain take a passive attitude towards their rehabilitation, they are depending on providers to take care of them. This is not as successful as when the person in pain takes an active role and engages in self-care. Remember, the doctor is the teacher. They must have a learner who wants to learn.

Behaviors. Behaviors are a range of actions made by individuals in combination with their environment. People who suffer from chronic pain engage is similar behaviors. Some people may use extended bed rest as a means of controlling their pain flare-up. Most adults sleep an average of 6–8 hours a night, which leaves 16 waking hours in the day. You must be moving more than half of that time. When people sit in the La-Z-Boy sofa, lie down on the couch, or sleep in bed during that time, that indicates they are not moving enough. They withdraw from activities of daily living and engage in irregular physical activity. Remember, if you are not moving and not sleeping, it is difficult to determine how you are going to feel better. You can read more about sleep hygiene in chapter 6 to help improve your sleep quality. Individuals with chronic pain will also self-medicate sometimes using other substances. It is important for them to realize that if the brain has a role in pain, then using illicit substances will only scramble the pain signals. You can read more about substances of abuse and their effects on the brain in chapter 2.

People who suffer from pain may also engage in fear-avoidance behaviors. They may develop chronic musculoskeletal pain as a result of avoidant behavior based on fear. If an individual experiences acute discomfort and delays addressing the situation by using avoidant behavior, a lack of pain increase reinforces this behavior. This may be why some people avoid normal activity, especially if their pain is of high intensity all the time. Avoidant behavior is healthy when encouraging the individual to avoid stressing injuries and permitting them to heal at the acute phase. However, it is harmful when discouraging the individual from activity after the injury is healed as in the chronic pain phase.

Family & Environment. Family is the universal institution where basic relationships exist. Family is the "first" reference group that shapes our world. There are profound effects of pain on family, and equally profound effect of family responses on their loved one's pain.

A Closer Look

What roles may be altered due to the pain sufferer?

Role reversals may emerge between the pain sufferer and other family members. Family members may have added employment responsibilities, but there are other roles that one should consider may have changed:

- Supportive husband/wife
- Mother/father
- Breadwinner
- Community volunteer
- Cook
- Gardener
- Chauffeur
- Errand runner

- Homework supervisor
- Social director
- Disciplinarian
- Confidant
- Bill payer
- Financial planner
- Active neighbor/friend
- Vacation planner/participant

There are two dimensions of chronic pain. There is the loved one whose pain does not show, has fluctuating activity levels, unpredictable mood swings, and lack of interest, loses support, and is isolating. Then there is the family who is unable to see or feel the pain, take on more responsibility, have added stress, lose plans and hopes, deal with emotional outbursts, and lose support.

Family may be responsible, in part, for maintaining and perpetuating pain problems. Those who surround the person manifesting pain behavior will be required to respond to them. Their mere presence may come to serve as a cue for increased reports of pain behavior. Reinforcement of maladaptive behavior may occur when family unintentionally provide attention or react caringly to pain complaint. Remember, attention is a form of love. This can best be seen in situations where the person in pain has an over-protective partner or spouse. Family members may also promote fear of harm. They often mean well but begin taking over tasks and even speaking for their loved one. The family member may perform task for the loved one in order to terminate the stressful impact of their complaints of pain. Family members may also take on more responsibilities which may detract from their loved one's independence and self-efficacy. Remember, it is important for the person suffering from pain to maintain their independence and that family support their attempts to return to work. Some families also deal with emotional problems at a somatic level. In other words, they exhibit their emotional problems with physical complaints. The opposite is also true. Some people who suffer from pain live alone, have no family nearby, or have no support system in place. They often feel ignored or express frustration because they do not have anyone to talk to about their problems.

Chronic pain can also impact the family system with significant negative consequences. Chronic pain intrudes on every aspect of family life. There may be loss of sexual expression and intimacy in couples. There may be social isolation which then enhances their involvement with the healthcare system. Family members may show evidence of depression or anxiety. They may engage in ongoing unexpressed family conflict or childhood family issues. Sometimes family members will begin to believe their pained loved one is attention-seeking or avoiding their responsibilities which will negatively impact their relationships.

Compensation & Work Issues. This is perhaps the most sensitive and complicated issue faced commonly by persons with chronic pain. For many people who have pain, the thought of returning to work seems unachievable because they already spent too much time off work. They worry how their pain may have a negative impact on their work ability due to the demands on the body. Some people may have been ineffective managing their pain at work in the past or were punished at work due to their pain. Since some people lack an incentive to return to work, they may pursue disability benefits or compensation claims. However, they may lack the historical documents outlining their pain or may have had their previous claims denied.

A Closer Look

What is the difference between a disability and a handicap?

In 1980, the World Health Organization (WHO) created the international classification of illness. They distinguished the differences between several words that people use interchangeable. Pathology is the underlying disease or diagnosis. Impairment is the immediate physiologic consequences, symptoms, and signs. Disability is the functional consequences or the abilities lost. Handicap is the social or societal consequences or the freedoms lost.

Pathology → Impairment → Disability → Handicap

This model was updated in 2012 by the International Classification of Functioning, Disability, and Health (ICF) model of disablement. This model further clarified each area and considered how environmental and personal factors come into play:

Health condition → Body functions → Activity → Participation

For Providers

As a provider, the goal is to keep people employed as long as they can work. As I mentioned before, work is very healthy. There may be several potential barriers to returning to work that may need to be addressed. The person may have some job-related fears or dissatisfaction with their employment. They may have fears of re-injury. You will need to identify psychosocial barriers to returning to work. There may be a need to reduce combative relationships between the person in pain and their employer. You will also need to identify and address workplace accommodations that may be barriers.

There are several accommodations that are common for people with chronic pain. These individuals will need to take frequent breaks, divide large assignments into smaller tasks, and engage in pacing as outlined in chapter 4.

Active vs. Passive Coping

People who suffer from chronic pain tend to seek out passive treatments versus active alternatives. They tend to go for short-term relief at a long-term cost. In pain management, active treatments should be the primary focus, with passive interventions as an adjunct, not the other way around. It is possible that the reason why people gravitate to passive treatments is because providers have reinforced that belief. Providers continue to use these passive treatments as the standard of care for chronic pain management.

Active treatments (such as home exercises, relaxation techniques, and mindfulness practices) can be available where and when the person needs to manage the pain. However, they rely on the person to actively participate in these techniques at home away from the clinic. In addition, active techniques have a synergistic rather than a mere additive effect when combined with other interventions. It has been theorized that the active approach offers the potential to change physical factors (such as pain) and psychological factors (such as self-efficacy). Past research has shown that active movement and behavioral treatments for chronic low back pain are generally effective.

Passive therapies (such as medications, interventions, and surgery) tend to be discouraged as a primary focus by scholars. Passive treatments have the potential of reinforcing feelings of powerlessness in people who suffer from chronic pain. They also put the responsibility for pain management back in the hands of the provider. Passive options require people to be a submissive recipient of treatment. Passive treatment can help with immediate pain relief, but active treatment keeps the individual functional in the long-term. For example, when someone undergoes a surgery and fails to follow a proper rehabilitation program, they may still have pain long after recovering from their operation. Many passive interventions have shown positive effects for acute low back pain. Interestingly, the interventions shown to be effective in acute pain appear less effective in chronic pain. It has been recommended that passive modalities not be employed except when necessary to facilitate participation in an active treatment program. While passive treatments can be successful, it is critical to shift the person into a model of active care.

A Closer Look

What are examples of active versus passive coping?

ACTIVE	PASSIVE
• Home exercises from physical therapy	• Medication management
• Self-hypnosis	• Interventional therapies
• Relaxation techniques	• Surgery
• Mindfulness practices	• Massage
• Adaptive recreation therapy activities	• Acupuncture
• Rehabilitation programs	• Healing touch
• Posture and body mechanics	• TENS unit
• Biofeedback	

It may be helpful to think of all the treatments covered in this book as existing in a continuum, with passive treatments being on one end and active on the other. In the middle, one could envision treatments as being "transitional." For example, a chiropractor may transition from using myofascial release to teaching the person exercises to do at home. This is so the patient is able to increase range of motion at home while still offering spinal manipulation. Thus, the chiropractor would rely on the person to actively participate in the techniques away from clinic. This is different from a massage therapist or acupuncturist who could teach someone else on how to perform the techniques, which would require the person to continue being a submissive recipient of the treatment from another person.

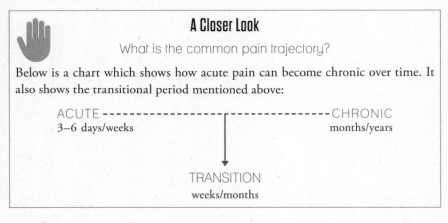

A Closer Look

What is the common pain trajectory?

Below is a chart which shows how acute pain can become chronic over time. It also shows the transitional period mentioned above:

ACUTE - CHRONIC
3–6 days/weeks   months/years

TRANSITION
weeks/months

Comparing Treatment Models

The rules about treating chronic pain have changed in the medical field in the past two decades. Remember, acute pain is pain lasting less than three to six months. Acute pain is directly related to tissue damage, is immediate, and usually of a short duration. The cause of acute pain can usually be diagnosed and treated. Acute pain is a symptom of an injury. When the injury heals, pain goes away! Providers tend to use the biomedical approach to treat acute pain. They use technology as its diagnostic strategy, are short-term in time span, assess cause, and define pain as a symptom which separates the body and mind.

Governing agencies have suggested that if pain persists beyond six months, or the normal time of healing, then the pain is chronic. The person in pain should then be approached using the "biopsychosocial" method. A biopsychosocial approach rewrites the rules and expectations about treatment. People who suffer from chronic pain are encouraged to take a more active role in their treatment. This is different from the biomedical approach used during the acute phase of pain. Active care can counter-stimulate the pain in the brain. It can teach the brain to move the relentless, persistent, and constant pain signaling to comfort and pleasure. It is recommended people move from a passive "disempowering" stance to a more active "empowering" stance.

A Closer Look

How are the biomedical and biopsychosocial models different?

Below is a chart showing how each model differs from the other.

	Biomedical	Biopsychosocial
Mind and body relationship	Body and mind separate	Holistic—"Total Person"
Pain defined as . . .	Symptom	Complex problem
Assessment goal . . .	Identify cause	Identify effects
Diagnostic strategy . . .	High techonology	Comprehensive psychosocial
Treatment goal . . .	Cure	Restoring function
Time span . . .	Short term—pain relief	Long term—reactivation
Provider role . . .	Expert	Teacher/coach
Patient role . . .	Passive/helpless	Active/responsible
More appropriate for . . .	Acute pain	Chronic pain

Chronification of Acute Pain

One of the more common questions I get asked is how an acute pain condition becomes a chronic pain condition. Typically, I like to refer to low back pain as an example. About 90% of low back pain cases will resolve on their own in about 6 weeks. Anywhere from 3% to 20% of acute low back pain cases develop into persistent pain. An additional 25% to 60% of acute cases will have a relapse 1 year after the initial episode. Unfortunately, there is not one single path to explain how some acute cases will become persistent. However, there are particular situations which have been shown to be related to the chronification of acute pain, including the following:

- There is a failure to respond to treatment in reasonable time.
- The initial injury is not as catastrophic.
- The level of disability is out of proportion with the degree of impairment.
- There is a history of adverse childhood events.
- There is evidence of fear-avoidance.
- They engage in catastrophizing behaviors.
- They have perceived injustices.

- They have psychological distress.
- They are affected by cultural factors (e.g. toxic work environment).
- They experience family influences.
- There are pending worker's compensation or personal injury actions.
- There is a family history of chronic pain.
- They are female and/or have a history of abuse.
- They experience effects of job type and work environment.
- They have low SES or educational status.
- They exhibit a maladaptive coping style.
- They have poor prior general health or functional status.

The next section is going to outline the treatment plans for specific pain conditions. Keep in mind that anyone can read a medical book to find the recommended treatments for any pain condition. It takes a more trained eye to recognize how lifestyle imbalances and coping styles can exacerbate any pain condition. When I train healthcare providers in chronic pain management, I often talk about using these viewpoints. They need to take several steps away from their patient and ask, "What is it about *this* person that brings them into my clinic compared to other people with this condition? What is it that *this* person needs to see improvement in their pain condition beyond the recommended treatments?"

Treatment Plans for Specific Pain Conditions

Cancer Pain

Most of the pain with cancer is from the cancer itself as it spreads to organs, bone, or nerves. Cancer treatments themselves can cause pain. Taking care of pain is important to quality of life for people with cancer and should be a part of good cancer care. Pain relief will help people with cancer feel stronger and better able to cope with their disease and its treatments.

Treatment Course: Pain associated with cancer can be relieved with medicine and other treatments outlined in this book. The frequency and intensity of the treatment is dependent on the prognosis. Specific cancer pain treatments are beyond the scope of this book.

Complex Regional Pain Syndrome

CRPS, also known as Reflex Sympathetic Dystrophy (RSD), is caused by abnormal activity in the sympathetic nervous system. This syndrome most often results from an injury or surgery to an extremity, particularly the hand or foot. As the injury or surgery heals, the pain persists, intensifies, and can spread. The skin around the affected area can change color and be cold to the touch. It is typically a burning, itching kind of pain, and almost any stimulus to the affected area is painful. There can also be changes to hair and nail growth patterns.

Treatment Course: The earlier CRPS is identified and treated, the better the response to treatment. It is usually treated first with medications and physical therapy. If these treatments do not bring relief, the next step may be a nerve block. Another treatment option for refractory pain includes spinal cord stimulation (SCS). See chapter 3 for more information about the SCS.

Facial Pain

Atypical facial pain is a chronic pain syndrome that encompasses a wide group of facial pain problems. Atypical facial pain can have many different causes but the symptoms are all similar. The symptoms include a burning, pinching, pulling, aching or cramping that occurs on one side of the face, often in the region of the trigeminal nerve. It can extend into the upper neck or back of the scalp. Facial pain is ongoing for atypical facial pain, with few, if any, periods of remission, and may be an early stage of trigeminal neuralgia.

Treatment Course: This kind of pain is difficult to diagnose and does not respond well to medication. Because of the side effects of medications and the limits to their success, people may choose to pursue neurosurgical interventions.

Failed Back Surgery Syndrome

The term "failed back surgery syndrome" is a misnomer. Often, the name of this diagnosis leaves people feeling as though something wrong happened during their surgery. Failed back surgery is diagnosed when back pain or leg pain recurs or persists following an otherwise successful back surgery. Repair and regeneration of nerves can sometimes result in abnormal signal transmissions, interpreted in the brain as pain following the initial trauma.

Treatment Course: Abnormal regeneration of the nerves in the affected area following back surgery may explain why repeated surgery for disc herniations sometimes fails to relieve pain. A treatment option for failed back surgery syndrome includes SCS.

Headaches

There are several different types of headaches, including cervicogenic, cluster, migraine, and tension types. Here is a brief summary of each type.

Cervicogenic. These headaches are generally due to a neck injury. Pain is caused by damaged neck joints, ligaments, muscles, or cervical discs, all of which have complex nerve endings. When these neck structures are injured, nerve endings send pain signals to the brain, intermingling with nerve fibers of the trigeminal nerve. People with cervicogenic headaches have the symptoms of tension headaches, but some may have the symptoms of migraine and cluster headaches.

Cluster. These headaches feel like an attack of excruciating, burning pain in an eye socket or surrounding area, lasting 15 to 180 minutes, recurring from once every other day to 8 times per day. There are characteristic symptoms that occur on the affected side of the face. These symptoms include a reddened eye, excessive tears, congested nostrils, drooping eyelid, smaller pupil size, and facial sweating.

Migraines. During an attack, changes in brain activity produce inflamed blood vessels and nerves around the brain causing a pulsating, throbbing pain. People who suffer from migraines may also experience nausea or vomiting and sensitivity to sound, light, or odors. A migraine is episodic, and often one-sided, occurring in the temple or forehead, behind the eye, or in the back of the head. The headache pain can last from a few hours to a few days and is often disabling.

Tension. These headaches are the most common form of headache. The pain is usually mild and can be alleviated by over the counter pain medications. It occurs on both sides of the head at the same time. Onset is slow and its duration varies, but it usually lasts less than a day.

Treatment Course: OTC and prescription medications may have a role in treatment or prevention. Medications combined with behavior therapies may be more effective. See chapter 4 for information about psychological interventions. In addition, alternative therapies aimed at stress reduction may help. They include meditation, massage and gentle neck stretches, rest in a quiet and dark room, hot or cold compresses to your head or neck, ingesting small amounts of caffeine, and the use of electrical stimulation as outlined in chapter 3.

Myofascial Pain Syndrome

Myofascial pain syndrome typically refers to localized and sometimes diffuse pain in the body due to skeletal muscle injury or strain. Muscle strains and injuries can lead to muscle spasms that restrict localized blood flow and thus oxygen delivery to the injured area. This can lead to the release of inflammatory chemicals in tissues that can sustain any localized muscle spasm. These spasmed areas can actually be felt under the skin as well as confined painful areas. Often, myofascial pain is secondary to some other primary problem restricting a person's motion.

Treatment Course: Typical treatment involves anti-inflammatory medications, physical therapy, and active stretching of the painful areas. Sometimes localized injections into the painful areas are required. Trigger point injections can refer pain outside of their localized areas.

Neuropathic Pain Syndromes

Neuropathy can come from prolonged pain that persists after an injury or without any obvious injury at all and is a dysfunction of nerves. Neuropathic pain results from a nervous system malfunction set off by nerve damage. That damage may have been caused by diseases such as diabetes, trauma, MS, shingles, syphilis, or medications (such as chemotherapy and HIV drugs). Rather than the nervous system functioning properly to signal presence of tissue injury, nerves themselves are malfunctioning and become the cause of pain. Some people experience a burning that makes wearing clothes and walking unbearable.

Treatment Course: Anticonvulsant and antidepressant drugs are often the first line of treatment. Some neuropathic pain studies suggest the use of non-steroidal anti-inflammatory drugs (NSAIDs). If another condition, such as diabetes, is involved, better management of that disorder may alleviate the pain. Other kinds of treatments can also help with neuropathic pain. Some of these include physical therapy, relaxation exercises, massage, and acupuncture as outlined in chapter 5. This syndrome responds poorly to standard pain treatment and may get worse instead of better over time.

Occipital Neuralgia

Occipital neuralgia is a chronic pain disorder caused by irritation or injury to occipital nerve located in the back of the scalp. Individuals with this disorder experience pain originating at the nape of the neck. Pain is described as throbbing and migraine-like, and spreads up and around the forehead and scalp. Occipital neuralgia can result from physical stress, trauma, or repeated contraction of muscles of the neck.

Treatment Course: The medical treatment for occipital neuralgia can vary. Often, conservative treatments including heat, massage, rest, physical therapy, muscle relaxants, and anti-inflammatory medications are used as first-line options. If the pain persists, daily medications to help calm the nerve may be used. Occipital nerve blocks using an injection of a local anesthetic and a steroid agent may be performed.

Pelvic Pain

Chronic pelvic pain is one of the most common pain problems affecting women. It may be a steady pain or a pain that comes and goes with the menstrual cycle. The pain may start with a physical problem that heals or seems to disappear, but pain continues because of changes in the nervous system or muscle tissues. The pain can affect the muscles of the abdomen, pelvis, urinary tract, and bowels, leading to changes in bowel and bladder function. The area's connective tissue and skin of the pelvic area may also become painful. Persistent pain can cause limited mobility, depression, and emotional problems. Causes can include, but are not limited to, endometriosis, pelvic congestion syndrome, muscle spasms, and cystitis.

Treatment Course: Depending on the cause, your doctor may recommend a number of medications to treat this condition. Other specific therapies or procedures may be added to the plan. These may include physical therapy, stretching exercises, massage, relaxation exercises, trigger point injections, neurostimulation, and psychotherapy. Sometimes your therapist will target specific points of pain using transcutaneous electrical nerve stimulation (TENS), which is outlined in chapter 3. Other times, your therapists will help you identify areas of tight muscles using biofeedback so that you can learn to relax those areas. See chapter 4 for more information about biofeedback. You may also want to consider Traditional Chinese Medicine techniques like acupuncture and moxibustion, summarized in chapter 5.

Phantom Limb Pain

Phantom limb pain is mild to extreme pain felt in the area where a limb has been amputated. Phantom limb sensations usually will disappear or decrease over time. Beyond six months, the prognosis for improvement is poor. Some people experience other sensations such as tingling, cramping, heat, and cold in the portion of the limb removed. Any sensation experienced prior to amputation may be experienced in phantom limb. Although the limb is no longer there, nerve endings at the site of amputation continue to send pain signals to the brain that make the brain think the limb is still there.

Treatment Course: Recommended treatments include heat, biofeedback, massage, injections/nerve blocks, surgery, physical therapy, a TENS unit, neurostimulation, and medications. Your therapist may also include mirror box therapy in your treatment plan.

A Closer Look

What is mirror box therapy?

A mirror box is a box with two mirrors in the center (one facing each way), and it was invented by Vilayanur S. Ramachandran. Mirror box therapy is a treatment of phantom limb pain, but it has also been used for complex regional pain syndrome, stroke rehabilitation, and for hand and foot rehabilitation following an injury or surgery. In a mirror box the person places the good limb into one side, and the residual limb into the other. The person then looks into the mirror on the side with the good limb and makes "mirror symmetric" movements. Because the subject is seeing the reflected image of the good hand moving, it appears as if the phantom limb is also moving. Through the use of this artificial visual feedback, it becomes possible for the person to "move" the phantom limb. People report feeling like they still have a functioning limb even if it has been amputated.

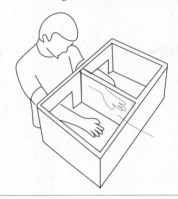

Post Herpetic Neuralgia

The herpes zoster, also called shingles, results from the reactivation of the same virus that causes chicken pox in children. Post-herpetic neuralgia is diagnosed when the pain from shingles does not go away. Only a small number of people with a shingles outbreak develop post-herpetic neuralgia. People over the age of 50 have a much higher incidence of persistent pain.

Treatment Course: No single treatment relieves post-herpetic neuralgia in all people. In many cases, it takes a combination of treatments to reduce the pain. These include lidocaine or capsaicin patches, anticonvulsants and antidepressants, and steroid injections. Sympathetic nerve blocks should be considered part of early treatment to help prevent post herpetic neuralgia. Antiviral medications have been found to help reduce or prevent the occurrence of post-herpetic neuralgia pain.

Post-Surgical Pain

More than 80% of people report pain after surgery, and 75% report the pain as moderate, severe, or even extreme. Post-surgical pain persists beyond the normal healing period and is not due to infection or any continuing surgical problem. Typically, it is due to prolonged avoidance of normal body motions causing secondary muscle shortening and spasms. It can also be due to the normal potential trauma of nerves that can occur with many surgeries. Most cases of postsurgical chronic pain are neuropathic.

Treatment Course: Oral medications should be taken over patient-controlled epidural analgesia (PCEA). PCEA is any method of allowing a person in pain to administer their own pain relief. The infusion is programmable by prescriber. If it is programmed and functioning as intended, the machine is unlikely to deliver an overdose of medication. Providers must always observe the first administration of any PCEA medication that has not already been administered by the provider to respond to allergic reactions.

Spasticity

Spasticity is a neurological condition that causes an abnormal increase in muscle tone, most often occurring when nerve pathways regulating muscles are damaged. Spasticity is a common complication of cerebral palsy, spinal cord injury, MS, stroke, and traumatic brain injuries. Resistant to the normal stretching that occurs during use, spastic muscles may remain abnormally contracted for long periods. Spasticity can lead to incoordination, loss of function, permanent muscle shortening, and repetitive muscle spasms. It can also be painful, as it may pull joints into abnormal positions and prevent full range of motion.

Treatment Course: Current spasticity management options include physical therapy, occupational therapy, aquatics, neurostimulation, biofeedback, taping, splints, wheelchairs, oral medications, botox injections, and surgical interventions like implanting intrathecal drug delivery systems filled with baclofen. See chapter 3 for more information about intrathecal drug delivery systems.

Trigeminal Neuralgia

Trigeminal neuralgia, also called tic duloreaux, is one of most intense pain syndromes, typically diagnosed in adults after age 50. It may be caused by compressive blood vessels, tumors, and vascular malformations, which result in an electric shock-like pain in areas of face where branches of nerve are distributed. These areas include the lips, eyes, nose, scalp, forehead, upper jaw, and lower jaw. The episode lasts only a few seconds, but the pain experienced can be excruciating. The disorder most often affects only one side of face, but some people experience pain on both sides at different times.

Treatment Course: To treat trigeminal neuralgia, your doctor usually will prescribe medications to lessen or block the pain signals sent to your brain. They may also recommend surgical options. However, some people have found improvement with treatments such as acupuncture, biofeedback, chiropractic, and vitamin or nutritional therapy. See chapter 6 for more information about nutritional therapies.

Fibromyalgia

10 million people in the US have fibromyalgia and 3% to 6% of the world. Fibromyalgia is a chronic pain syndrome characterized by widespread musculoskeletal pain, multiple tender points, and fatigue. A person is considered to have fibromyalgia if they have widespread pain in combination with tenderness

in at least 11 of 18 specific tender point sites, with these symptoms persisting for more than three months. People with this disorder may also experience other symptoms including sleep disturbances, morning stiffness, irritable bowel syndrome, and anxiety. Most people with fibromyalgia describe their pain as aching all over, as if their muscles have been pulled or overworked. Sometimes their muscles twitch and at other times they burn. Diagnosis is made by history and physical exam with your doctor. Fibromyalgia is marked by hypersensitivity and sensory amplification. Fibromyalgia is also considered a functional somatic syndrome.

Treatment Course: When it comes to fibromyalgia treatments, there are drugs, alternative remedies, and lifestyle habits that may help decrease pain and improve sleep. See chapter 6 for a review of lifestyle imbalance management. Your treatment plan will also include physical therapy, moist heat, regular aerobic exercise, relaxation, acupuncture, hypnosis, and other psychological interventions to help you self-manage your symptoms.

A Closer Look

What are functional somatic syndromes?

Fibromyalgia is a type of functional somatic syndrome which is a diagnosis of central sensitization. The term functional somatic syndrome refers to several related syndromes that are characterized by symptoms, suffering, and disability. This is instead of disease-specific, demonstrable abnormalities of structure or function. Each medical specialty has their own "dumpster" diagnosis.

Functional Somatic Syndromes by Speciality

Gastroenterology	Irritable bowel syndrome, non-ulcer dyspepsia
Gynecology	Premenstrual syndrome, chronic pelvic pain
Rheumatology	Fibromyalgia
Cardiology	Atypical or non-cardiac chest pain
Respiratory medicine	Hyperventilation syndrome
Infectious diseases	Chronic (postviral) fatigue syndrome
Neurology	Tension headache
Dentistry	Temporomandibular joint dysfunction, atypical facial pain
Ear, nose, and throat	Globus syndrome
Allergy	Multiple chemical sensitivity

There are four psychosocial factors that propel this cycle of symptom amplification:

1. The belief that you have a serious disease

---

2. The expectation that your condition is likely to worsen
3. The "sick role," including the effects of litigation and compensation
4. The alarming portrayal of the condition as catastrophic and disabling

People who suffer from these conditions will report feeling like they are "falling apart." I often will ask these people what the treatment is for syndromes such as fibromyalgia. Their response is usually something like "Lyrica." That is incorrect! The number one treatment for these conditions is actually education and movement.

Pediatric Pain

At least 15% of children have some type of pain. There are more girls than boys who have pain, but again that may be because women seek treatment for pain more than men. The most common pain complaints among children are headaches, abdominal pain, and musculoskeletal pain. These conditions lead to physical disability, anxiety, sleep disturbance, school absence, social withdrawal, severe parenting stress, and dysfunctional family roles.

Treatment Course: These conditions can be managed effectively by a family doctor or may not require any professional attention. The path to chronicity is characterized by failed attempts to adjust and cope. It is important to remember that research on medications is based usually on adult data, so there is limited evidence in children. There is some good evidence for psychological interventions, but you should consider related factors. These factors include the child's temperament, parenting style, individual and familial coping strategies, previous pain experiences, fitness and activity levels, and socioeconomic environment.

Geriatric Pain

As we age, the incidence and prevalence of certain pain syndromes will increase. However, if someone who is 80 years old never complains of pain and starts today, then this may not be age-related. Pain is typically underreported amongst our oldest old, as it is believed that pain is a normal process of aging. The elderly present with increased fat mass, decreased muscle mass, and decreased body water, all of which have important consequences on drug distribution. It is also important to beware of the toxic reactions of medications in this age group. One must also consider sensory limitations when working with this population. You may want to provide written instructions in large print, allow for extra time, and amplify audio.

Treatment Course: A multidisciplinary approach is recommended to investigate all possible options for pain management, including medications, interventional procedures, physical rehabilitation, and psychological support.

Burnout

Burnout is a term created by Freudenberger in 1974. It is the increased feelings of emotional exhaustion, an impersonal response towards others, and dissatisfaction with work accomplishments. Burnout is not a simple result of long hours. The pessimism, depression, and exhaustion of burnout can occur when you're not in control of how you carry out your responsibilities. It can occur when you're working toward goals that don't resonate with you and when you lack social support. Burnout occurs among people with pain, caregivers, and medical professionals. In fact, between 10% and 70% of nurses, and 30% and 50% of physicians, suffer from burnout. The specialty of medicine with the most burnout is emergency medicine, and the one with the least amount of burnout is dermatology. Research has shown that about 54% of physicians show one sign of burnout. These signs include

- emotional exhaustion
- depersonalization
- low personal accomplishment
- early retirement
- job changes
- more medical malpractice suits
- depression and/or anxiety
- suicidal ideation
- increased absenteeism
- increased alcohol use
- problems with relationships, including divorce

All of these signs are harmful, but the one that is most concerning is that burnout also harms others for which we care. It can lead to

- lack of professionalism
- increased risk of errors
- ordering unnecessary tests and procedures
- decreased quality of care

A Closer Look

How does your burnout harm others?

People who are experiencing burnout can have a negative impact on those around them, both by causing greater personal conflict and by disrupting tasks. You can learn a lot about how to address burnout from airline inflight announcements. How many times have you heard the flight attendant say, "If the cabin air pressure changes dramatically, oxygen masks might fall from the ceiling directly in front of you. If a child is seated beside you, put on your own mask before helping to put a mask on the child." The same tactic should be used in self-care. You must address your own needs before you can attend to the needs of those around you. You can do this by using some of the techniques reviewed in chapter 4 on psychological interventions. You can also use some of the strategies for coping that follow. Remember, self-care is important for you to keep functioning optimally. For example, you wouldn't go to the dentist twice a year and never clean your teeth, would you?

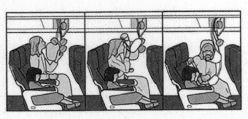

There are several causes of burnout, including personal, job, and organizational characteristics:

- Personal: sociodemographic variables, self-efficacy, and social support
- Job: relationships, role conflicts, role ambiguity, and role overload
- Organizational: how rewards and punishments are linked to performance

There are several recommendations to reduce burnout in your life:

- Set boundaries (as discussed in chapter 7)
- Take control when possible
- Engage with friends, family, and community
- Exercise regularly
- Practice stress management techniques (covered in chapter 4)
- Reorganize your commitments
- Reduce hassles
- Get enough quality sleep (as discussed in chapter 6)
- Seek professional help
- Practice gratitude
- Enhance resilience

A Closer Look

How do I know If I am burned out?

There are physical symptoms, behaviors, thoughts and feelings related to burnout. The table below shows a summary of symptoms for your reference.

Physical Symptoms	Behaviors	Thoughts/Emotions
· Exhaustion · Chronic fatigue · Headaches · Gastrointestinal issues · Sleep disorders · Muscular tension · Vulnerability to illness · Lingering illness	· Irritability · Anger · Resentment · Isolation · Relationship problems · Rigid thinking · Self-righteousness · Increased drug use	· Emotional numbness · Hypersensitivity · Cynicism · Apathy · Helplessness · Hopelessness · Depression · Overidentification with people who are sick

The following section outlines several strategies for general pain coping that you can use to combat burnout, such as resilience, distraction, social support, and goal setting.

Strategies for Coping

Resilience

Resilience is the process of adapting well in the face of adversity, trauma, tragedy, threats, or stress. Resilience is the ability to maintain successful outcomes or recover in response to a stressor. Resilient individuals are best described as having high levels of pain, but low interference/emotional burden. In fact, about 37% of people reporting high pain intensity have low pain disability. Resilient individuals have more adaptive pain coping, lower catastrophizing, decreased use of prescription pain medication, and decreased healthcare utilization. Resilience factors positively influence pain outcomes. There are several environmental and internal sources of resilience, including:

Environmental

- Family
- Friends
- Social support
- Community
- Resources
- Culture

Internal

- Cognitive/emotional (such as hope and psychological flexibility)
- Personality (such as optimism and extroversion)

- Physical/Behavioral (such as sleep quality and fitness)
- Existential/Spiritual (such as acceptance and life purpose)

Resilience-based approaches yield benefits in pain and psychological functioning. Developing resilience is a personal journey. Note that an approach to building resilience that works for one person might not work for another. Examples of resilience-based approaches include:

- Random acts of kindness
- Counting your blessings
- Expressing gratitude
- Cherishing positive experiences
- Nurturing humor
- Practicing forgiveness
- Creating meaning in your life
- Loving kindness meditation

Some or many of the ways to build resilience may be appropriate to consider in developing your own personal strategy.

Distraction

Distraction is the process of diverting the attention of an individual or group from a desired area of focus and thereby blocking or diminishing the reception of undesired information. In this case, the undesired information are the pain signals. Distraction requires the mental capacity to concentrate and the physical ability/ energy to engage in distracting activities. There are several examples of activities used for distractions, including

- Using appropriate humor
- Playing music
- Listening to audio books
- Making jewelry or other crafts
- Counting forward or backward
- Deep breathing
- Blowing bubbles
- Reciting the alphabet
- Reading or writing
- Tapping fingers
- Drawing, doodling, coloring, or doing puzzles
- Watching TV or DVDs
- Taking a mindful walk

Distraction is useful for brief pain episodes. An example is when undergoing procedural pain, such as needle sticks. Keep in mind that the awareness of the pain may return once the distraction ends. The distraction is more successful if you choose something you are interested in. The activity must stimulate the major senses (hearing, sight, touch, movement, and so on) in order to be engaging. You also want the potential to increase the distraction stimulus when your pain increases. An example is when beating a drum or creating music as covered in chapter 6.

Social Support

Social support is the perception and actuality that one is cared for, has assistance available from other people, and that one is part of a supportive social network. These supportive resources can be emotional, tangible, informational, companionship, and/or intangible, like personal advice. Social support can be obtained from a group or an individual. This person or persons allow you to express feelings about pain or tell your story, provide encouragement and reassurance, and discuss your problems or other concerns. Support can come from many sources, such as family, friends, pets, neighbors, coworkers, organizations, and so on. You can also obtain support from a referral to a psychologist, social worker, or clergy as necessary. Government-provided social support is often referred to as public aid.

A Closer Look

Where can I find a social support group in my area?

There is an amazing resource available to people who suffer from chronic pain. This is the American Chronic Pain Association (ACPA) website: theacpa.org. The mission of the ACPA is to facilitate peer support and education for individuals with chronic pain and their families, and to raise awareness among the health care community, policy makers, and the public at large about issues of living with chronic pain.

The ACPA was founded in 1980 by Ms. Penney Cowan in Pittsburgh, Pennsylvania. After many years of living with chronic pain, Penney had taken part in a pain management program and was eager to maintain the skills she had learned there when she returned to her daily life. She reached out to members of her community and created the first ACPA support group. Today several hundred ACPA support groups meet across the United States, Canada, Great Britain, and many other countries. The ACPA's unique materials are a primary resource for individuals seeking to improve the quality of their lives and for the professionals who help them.

Intimacy is healing. Intimacy is a close, familiar, and usually affectionate or loving personal relationship with another person or group. There are different types of intimacy and each one can nourish you.

- Being emotionally intimate with someone means that you can talk to them about your innermost thoughts. It includes emotional expressions such as compassion and forgiveness.
- Intellectual intimacy includes exchanging ideas and thoughts about things you think and care about.

- Physical intimacy is not only sexual or erotic. It also is being affectionate with someone, which can include everything from hugging to holding hands to kissing to cuddling on the couch.
- Experiential intimacy may include taking a walk, biking, seeing a movie, or even sitting in a garden. It can also include activities such as public service, altruism, and being part of a community.
- Spiritual intimacy is sharing awe-inspiring moments with someone. It may include spirituality, religion, prayer or meditation, exploring nature of the arts, or working with a traditional healer. See chapter 6 for more information about spirituality.

Setting Goals

Living life to the fullest is one of the most common goals. Some people might say that humans put all their effort towards setting and achieving goals. Goals are part of every aspect of life. It is something by which we measure and motivate ourselves. However, figuring out how to do it is a conundrum that has challenged so many people throughout the ages. It may not be a complex problem after all. Everything comes down to priorities, whether you make a conscious choice or go with subconscious preferences. Without setting goals, life becomes disordered and you would lose control. Treat your life as a gift, appreciate every little thing, and develop a sense of purpose. Develop a convincing and fulfilling reason to get out of bed and to keep going. Florence Nightingale once said:

"Live life when you have it. Life is a splendid gift—there is nothing small about it."

Instead of vague resolutions, S.M.A.R.T. goal setting brings structure and a way to track your goals. The acronym S.M.A.R.T. can be used to provide a more comprehensive definition of goal setting:

- **S: Specific goals**
  - » are well defined
  - » are clear to anyone that has a basic knowledge of the situation
- **M: Measurable goals**
  - » help you know if the goal is obtainable and how far away from completion
  - » help you find out when you have achieved your goal
- **A: Attainable goals**
  - » foster agreement with all involved what the goals should be
- **R: Realistic goals**
  - » are within the availability of resources, knowledge and time

- **T: Timely goals**
  - » provide enough time to achieve the goal
  - » don't provide too much time, which can affect performance

One way to start using S.M.A.R.T. goals in your pain management is to have a discussion with your primary provider about what you have learned in this book and how you would like to start exploring some of the options outlined.

Conclusion

The final chapter reviewed different ways to cope with chronic pain. The goals of this book were to provide you with education about chronic pain and to review the available assessments and treatments. These are the cornerstones for pain management. I hope that after you read this book, you will implement some of what you learned and discuss some of these points with your primary care provider. In this way, you will be an active participant in your care and will witness more success in this endeavor.

References

ACC. The New Zealand acute low back pain guide and assessing yellow flags in acute low back pain: Risk factors for long-term disability and work loss. New Zealand Guideline Group; 2003.

Afari, N., Ahumada, S., Wright, L., et al. (2014). Psychological Trauma and Functional Somatic Syndromes: A Systematic Review and Meta-Analysis. *Psychosomatic Medicine*, 76, 2–11.

Agency for Clinical Innovation. (2018). Pain Management Network. Segment 4 - How can distraction be used to manage pain? Available at: https://www.aci.health.nsw.gov.au/ chronic-pain/painbytes/ pain-and-mind-body-connection/how-can-distraction-be-used-to-manage-pain.

Aktivortho. Solutions-Passive vs. active therapy. Available at: http://www.aktivortho. com/solution-passive-active-therapy.asp.

American Chronic Pain Association. (2018). American Chronic Pain Association: About us. Available at: https://theacpa.org/About-Us.

Anderson B. Randomized clinical trial comparing active versus passive approaches to the treatment of recurrent and chronic low back pain. Dissertation for the University of Miami; 2005.

Arnold, L., Hudson, J, Keck, P., Auchenbach, M., Javaras, K., & Hess, E. (2006). Comorbidity of firbomyalgia and psychiatric disorders. *Clinical Psychiatry*, 67 (8), 1219–25.

Arnold, L., Keck, P., & Welge, J. (2000). Antidepressant treatment of fibromyalgia: A meta-analysis and review. *Psychosomatics*, 41, 104–13.

Arnstein P. Clinical coach for effective pain management. F.A. Davis Company: Philadelphia, PA; 2010.

Aure O, Nilsen J, Vasseljen O. Manual therapy and exercise therapy in patients with chronic low back pain: A randomized, controlled trial with 1-year follow-up. *Spine*, 2003; 28: 525–531.

Baldwin C, Long K, Kroesen, K. A profile of military veterans in the southwestern US who use complementary and alternative medicine: Implications for integrated care. *JAMA Intern Med*, 2002; 12: 1697–1704.

Barsky, A. & Borus, J. (1999). Functional Somatic Syndromes. *Ann Intern Med*, 130, 910–921.

Bode G. Chiropractic . . . Active vs. passive care it makes all the difference in the world. Available at: http:// bodechiropractic. blogspot.com/2010/11/chiropractic-active-vs-passive-care-it.html.

Cordes, C. & Doughtery, T. (1993). A review and an integration of research on job burnout. *Acad Manage Rev*, 18, 621–656.

Cowen, P. (1998). *Family manual: A manual for families of persons with pain*. American Chronic Pain Association.

Elliott, A., Burton, C., & Hannaford, P. (2014). Resilience does matter: Evidence from a 10-year cohort record linkage study. *BMJ Open*, 4, e003917.

Ferrell B, Rhiner M, Ferrell B. Development and implementation of a pain education program. *Cancer* 1993; 72: 3426–3432.

Flor H, Braun C, Elbert T, Birbaumer N. Extensive reorganization of primary somatosensory cortex in chronic back pain patients. *Neurosci Lett* 1997; 224: 5–8.

Flor, H., Turk, D. & Rudy, T. (1987). Pain and families. II. Assessment and treatment. *Pain*, 30, 29–45.

Freudenberger, H. (1974). Staff burnout. *J Social Issues*, 30, 159–185.

Garcia, H., McGeary, D., McGeary, C., & Finley, E. (2014). Burnout in Veterans Health Administration Mental Health Providers in Posttraumatic Stress Clinics. *Psychological Services*, 11, 50–59.

Grant, M. (2013). Ten tips for communicating with a person suffering from chronic pain. Overcoming Pain Website. Available at: www.overcomingpain.com

Haas M, Groupp E, Kraemer D. Dose-response for chiropractic care of chronic low back pain. *Spine*, 2004; 4: 574–583.

Hassett, A. & Finan, P. (2016). The role of resilience in the clinical management of chronic pain. *Curr Pain Headache Rep*, 20, 39.

Hsiao A, Wong M, Goldstein M, et al. Variation in complementary and alternative medicine (CAM) use across racial/ethnic groups and the development of ethnic-specific measures of CAM use. *J Altern Complement Med*, 2006; 12: 281–290.

Kannerstein, D. & Whitman, S. (2007). Surviving a loved one's chronic pain. *Practical Pain Management*, January/February, 49–52.

Karoly, P. & Ruehlman, L. (2006). Psychological "resilience" and its correlates in chronic pain: Findings from a national community sample. *Pain*, 123, 90–97.

Keller A, Hayden J, Bombardier C, van Tulder M. Effect sizes of non-surgical treatments of non-specific low-back pain. *Eur Spine J*, 2007; 16: 1776–1788.

Kralik D, Koch T, Price K, Howard N. Chronic illness self-management: Taking action to create order. *J Clin Nurs*, 2004; 13: 259–267.

Krasner, M., Epstein, R., Beckman, H., et al. (2009). Association of an educational program in mindful communication with empathy and attitudes among primary care physicians. *JAMA*, 1284–1293.

Kroesen K, Baldwin C, Brooks A, et al. US military veterans' perceptions of the conventional medical care system and their use of complementary and alternative medicine. *Fam Pract*, 2002; 19: 57–64.

Lewandowski, W., Morris, R., Draucker, C. & Risko, J. (2007). Chronic pain and the family: Theory-driven treatment approaches. *Issues in Mental Health Nursing*, 28, 1019–1044.

Loranger L. Good practice: Active vs. passive treatments. Physiotherapy Alberta News. Available at: https://www.physiotherapyalberta.ca/physiotherapists/news/good_practice_active_vs._passive_treatments?page=12.

Mannion A, Muntener M, Taimela S, Dvorak J. A randomized clinical trial of three active therapies for chronic low back pain. *Spine* 1999; 24: 2435–2448.

Maslach, C., Jackson, S., & Letter, M. (1996). *Maslach Burnout Inventory Manual, 3rd ed.* Palo Alto: CA. Consulting Psychologists Press.

Miller, D. (1995). Stress and burnout among health-care staff working with people affected by HIV. *Br J Guid Counc*, 23, 19–32.

Moskowitz M, Golden M. *Neuroplastix: Change the brain; Relieve the pain; Transform the person.* Available at: http://www.neuro plastix.com/styled-6/styled-7/introduction.html.

Nicassio, P. & Radojevic, V. (1993). Models of family functioning and their contribution to patient outcomes in chronic pain. *Motivation & Emotion*, 17, 295–316.

Pergolizzi, J., Raffa, R., & Taylor, R. (2014). Treating acute pain in light of the chronification of pain. *Pain Manag Nurs*, 15(1), 380–90.

Reflex Pain Management. (2017). *Mirror Box Therapy That Works*. Available at: https://mirrorboxtherapy.com/.

Reitman C, Esses S. Conservative options in the management of spinal disorders, Part I. Bed rest, mechanical, and energy-transfer therapies. *Am J Orthop*, 1995; 24: 109–116.

Sigsbee, B. & Bernat, J. (2014). Physician burnout: A neurologic crisis. *Neurology*, 83, 2302–2306.

Silver, J. (2004). *Chronic pain and the family*. Harvard University Press: Cambridge, MA.

Sood, A. Prasad, K., Schroeder, D., & Varkey, P. (2011). Stress management and resilience training among Department of Medicine faculty: A pilot randomized clinical trial. *J Gen Intern Med*, 26, 858–861.

Stinson J, White M, Isaac L, et al. Understanding the information and service needs of young adults with chronic pain: Perspectives of young adults and their providers. *Clin J Pain* 2013; 29: 600–612.

Tartakovsky, M. (2015). Nourishing the Different Types of Intimacy in Your Relationship. *Psychcentral: World of Psychology*. Available at: https://psychcentral.com/blog/nourishing-the-different-types-of-intimacy-in-your-relationship/.

Tripler Army Medical Center. (2016). Pain Syndromes. Website.

Turk D, Wilson H, Cahana A. Treatment of chronic non-cancer pain. *Lancet*, 2011; 377: 2226–2235.

University of Texas, School of Nursing, Family Nurse Practitioner Program. (2009). Management of fibromyalgia syndrome in adults. Austin, TX: University of Texas, School of Nursing; 1–14.

van Tulder M, Koes B, Bouter L. Conservative treatment of acute and chronic nonspecific low back pain: A systematic review of randomized controlled trials of the most common interventions. *Spine*, 1997; 22: 2128–2156.

van Tulder M, Ostelo R, Vlaeyen J, Linton S, Morley S, Assendelft W. Behavioral treatment for chronic low back pain: A systematic review within the framework of the Cochrane Back Review Group. *Spine*, 2000; 25: 2688–2699.

VHA Complementary & Integrative Health Services (formerly CAM). Healthcare Analysis & Information Group (HAIG). Washington, DC. Available at: http://vaww.va.gov/ HAIG/haig_pubs3_CAM.asp.

Wallace, J., Lemaire, J., & Ghali, W. (2009). Physician wellness: A missing quality indicator. *Lancet*, 374, 1714–1721.

Wessely, S. & White, P. (2004). There is only one functional somatic syndrome. *The British Journal of Psychiatry*, 185, 95–96.

Wessely, S., Nimnuan, C., & Sharpe, M. (1999). Functional somatic syndromes: One or many? *Lancet*, 354, 936–939.

Your Coach. (2018). SMART goals. Available at: http://www.yourcoach.be/en/coaching-tools/smart-goal-setting.php.

Acknowledgments

I would like to thank my father and mother for everything that they have done for me. Without you I am nothing. I want to thank my brother and my sister-in-law, who have always been my best friends and constant sources of support. I also want to thank my grandmother, who helped raise me and taught me to work hard for what I want.

I want to give a special thanks to all the veterans and providers who contributed to my education about chronic pain. I especially want to thank Carole Lexing, CRT; Chaplain R. Wayne Bearden, Jr., DMin, PhD; David Schaefer, DO; Dawn Dudek, LCSW; Eric Proescher, PsyD; Erica Lin, PharmD, BCACP; Erin Rule-Miller, CTRS; Felix Angelov, MD; Glenn Shalton, MA; Grant White, PhD; Jeffrey Albaugh, PhD, APRN, CUCNS; Julie Seltzer, OTD, OTR/L; Lynne O'Donnell, RN-MSN, ANP-BC, HTPA; Martina Moore, LAc; Rollin Socha, PhD; Sarah Catanese, PhD; Socrates Capili, PT; Susan Payvar, PhD, BCIA-C; Tracy Schafer, PsyD; and Valerie Carr, RD, for their contributions to this book.

About the Author

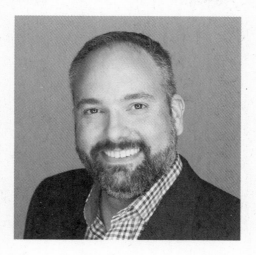

David Cosio, PhD, ABPP, has been the psychologist in the pain clinic and the CARF-accredited, interdisciplinary pain program at the Jesse Brown VA Medical Center in Chicago for nearly ten years. There, he provides consultative, educational, biofeedback, hypnosis, and a wide range of psychotherapeutic services. He also provides screening, assessment, diagnosis, and treatment of pain patients with co-occuring depressive, anxiety-related, substance-use disorders, and other mental health conditions, with an emphasis on the application of time-limited, evidence-based approaches (cognitive-behavioral therapy and acceptance & commitment therapy). He also serves as a faculty member of the University of Illinois–Chicago Pain Management Fellowship Program and a lecturer in the Department of Psychiatry at Northwestern University. He achieved specialist certi cation in Clinical Health Psychology by the American Board of Professional Psychology in 2017. Dr. Cosio received his PhD from Ohio University with a specialization in Health Psychology in 2008. He completed a behavioral medicine internship at the University of Massachusetts–Amherst Mental Health Services in 2008 providing care for UMass–Amherst students, their dependents, faculty and staff, and state employees of the greater Amherst area. He then completed a postdoctoral fellowship at the Edward Hines Jr. VA Hospital in 2009. There, he provided biopsychosocial-oriented care to patients in primary medical care settings, including primary care in the general medicine clinic and specialty clinics.

Dr. Cosio has done several presentations in health psychology at the regional level, such as the Midwest Pain Society and Society of Behavioral Medicine, and the national level, such as the American Pain Society and PainWeek. He has also published several articles on health psychology, specifically in the area of patient and provider pain education.

Scan to visit

drdavidcosio.com